The Ideas and Influence of Alan Williams

The Ideas and Influence of Alan Williams

BE REASONABLE – DO IT MY WAY!

Edited by

ANNE MASON
Research Fellow, Centre for Health Economics
University of York

and

ADRIAN TOWSE
Director, Office of Health Economics

Office of Health Economics

Radcliffe Publishing
Oxford • New York

Radcliffe Publishing Ltd
18 Marcham Road
Abingdon
Oxon OX14 1AA
United Kingdom

www.radcliffe-oxford.com

Electronic catalogue and worldwide online ordering facility.

British Library Cataloguing in Publication Data

A catalogue record for this book is available from the British Library.

ISBN-13: 978 184619 231 9

Typeset by Pindar New Zealand (Egan Reid), Auckland, New Zealand
Printed and bound by TJI Digital, Padstow, Cornwall, UK

Contents

Preface

Be reasonable: do it my way!

The sign on Alan Williams' desk revealed his sense of humour, a man who invited and relished debate, but always recognising that intellectual pursuits were a means to a practical end.

Alan was a man of principles: as Bob Sudgen notes, Alan was not interested in 'cookbook' economics, but in developing guiding principles that embraced and encouraged active intellectual engagement and development. Many of the authors of the papers contained within this book testify to their encounters with Alan – their intellectual journeys: Bob Sugden recalls his student days and attributes his chosen career path to Alan's influence; Ben van Hout reminisces about the impact Alan had upon Dutch efforts to develop quality of life measures; Bengt Jönsson echoes these sentiments, remembering how Alan's courageous intellectual battles within Europe paved the way for younger academics; and Alan Maynard reminds us of the debate that raged (and perhaps rages still) between egalitarians and libertarians, both parties guilty, Williams observed, of comparing the *ideal* characteristics of their own ideology with the *actual* characteristics of the opposing ideology. As intellectual journeys criss-crossed, new ideas were born and principles were refined or revised; for Alan, principles were never meant to be followed slavishly or unthinkingly.

However, Alan was also a practical man: intellectual debates were not an end in themselves, but were for the purpose of tackling real-world issues. He wanted to help decision makers engage with the issues facing them; the role of the health economist, as he saw it, was to provide a clear framework through which important factors informing the decision-making process were made accessible and transparent. Thus Alan continued, well into his retirement, to propound applications for his work: always an egalitarian, he argued that there were equity grounds for discriminating against older people who had had their 'fair innings' and that these grounds had important implications for the way in which scare resources were allocated within tightly squeezed healthcare budgets. In recent years, Alan worked with Aki Tsuchiya on broader issues of equity and fairness, exploring the implications of discriminating on the basis of gender or of socio-economic status.

Alan will perhaps best be remembered for his work within cost–benefit analysis. The quality-adjusted life year (QALY), born of his desire to find a generic outcome measure that would enable an assessment of the opportunity costs of healthcare interventions, synthesised the principled and the practical: life years added by a health intervention, adjusted for the quality of that life – not an end in itself but a means to achieving equitable health outcomes for all in the real world of limited resources. The role of the QALY as a tool for decision makers, enabling them to break out of the artificial constraints of 'welfarist' or 'Paretian' approaches, is discussed by Tony Culyer who sets out the key dividing points between Paretian and decision-making approaches to the application of economics in the allocation of resources in health care.

Within the healthcare sector, debates over the derivation and application of the QALY continue. Paul Kind reminds us that the quality element ('Q') of the QALY is critical: whose values should be used, how should values be combined and who should decide these issues? Kind argues that scope remains for methodological development, and that failure to address this has serious practical implications. Bob Sugden echoes these sentiments, questioning whether decision makers should decide, on behalf of the community, what the collective objective should be. Alan Maynard focuses on failure of healthcare systems to measure treatment effects, and advocates a system-wide application of patient-related outcomes measures (PROMs) as a way forward.

Alan's work on the QALYs also inspired methodological work on outcome measurement in other fields. Paul Dolan and Aki Tsuchiya's work on quality of life measurement in crime is in its early stages of development, with the SALY (safety-adjusted life year) proposed as a tool for measuring public safety. Their discussant, Martin Buxton, discusses the potential for a 'super-QALY' to embrace outcome measurement across different parts of the public sector, or even across multiple sectors.

Alan vigorously contested charges that cost–benefit analysis was a 'pseudo-science'. However, modern economic evaluation is not immune to the same allegations. Peggy and Richard Musgrave, who open this book with a tribute to Alan, reflect on his concern with the philosophical and ethical issues that underpin decision making, issues that must still be faced. To recognise and appreciate Alan's legacy, the task falls to the health economics community to ensure that we do not shirk our responsibilities: the need to be intellectually rigorous without being rigid; to keep in sight the practical implications of our work; to acknowledge the shortcomings within our discipline; and to move forward in the spirit of the Williams' way.

Anne Mason, Research Fellow, University of York
Adrian Towse, Director, Office of Health Economics, London
September 2007

List of contributors

Richard A Musgrave
HH Burbank Professor of Economics, Emeritus
Harvard University

Richard Abel Musgrave died on 15 January 2007 in Santa Cruz, California at the age of 96. A leading fiscal economist, he played a central role in shaping the modern field of public finance.

Peggy B Musgrave
Professor of Economics, Emerita
University of California, Santa Cruz

Robert Sugden
Professor of Economics
University of East Anglia, UK

Bengt Jönsson
Professor of Health Economics
Stockholm School of Economics, Sweden

Alan Maynard
Professor of Health Economics
University of York, UK

Dominique Polton
Directrice de la Stratégie des Études et des Statistiques
Caisse Nationale de l'Assurance Maladie, France

Anthony J Culyer
Professor of Economics, University of York, UK
Senior Scientist, Institute for Work & Health, Canada

Adrian Towse
Professor of Economics and Director
Office of Health Economics, London, UK

Aki Tsuchiya
Reader in Economics and Health Economics
University of Sheffield, UK

Paul Dolan
Professor of Economics
Imperial College London, UK

Jan Abel Olsen
Professor of Health Economics
University of Tromsø and University of Oslo, Norway

Paul Kind
Professor of Health Economics
University of York, UK

Ben van Hout
Professor of Medical Technology Assessment, University of Utrecht
The Netherlands and Scientific Director, Pharmerit

Martin Buxton
Professor of Health Economics and Director of the Health Economics Research Group
Brunel University, UK

CHAPTER 1

A tribute to our friend and colleague, Alan Williams

... Richard and Peggy Musgrave

We take the occasion of Alan's Memorial Conference to add our own words of esteem. Over the decades we travelled similar paths, both as colleagues and as friends. As colleagues, we shared fascination with the mysteries of 'public finance' and its powers to improve the world around us. As friends, we shared many visits, conferences and associations, crossing the Atlantic from east and west, from Vermont in the US to York in the UK. Hiking along the Pacific and in Vermont's green hills, we recall Alan's buoyant spirit, his gentle sense of humour spiced with sharp wit, a view of the world where not all was for the best, but neither was it beyond repair. Alan, striding firmly ahead, followed by June, slightly amused and with a twinkle of her own.

Alan's earlier work, as did ours, focused on the basics of fiscal theory, the nature of public goods, the intractable issues of equity and the ways of implanting fiscal functions into the various forms of governmental organisation, central and local, unitary and federal. Later on, focus shifted to policy issues and it is here that Alan's choice of health economics would lead him to his outstanding contributions, containing thoughts and directions which now enrich the papers of this conference.

Alan's turn to health economics was indeed a brilliant move, guided by his knack for combining analytical insights with a sense for practical application; to clear the ground first, before proceeding to more complex aspects. The purpose of health policy and research, as he saw it, is to improve the state of health of particular individuals, of groups and of nations, an essential ingredient of human well-being. Evaluation and comparison require measurement, a key issue to which Alan made one of his major contributions. The state of health as a policy concern has to be measured over time, traditionally done with reference to life expectation. Beginning with life expectancy as the point of departure, Alan then refined the concept, adding a human touch by allowing for the quality of life that was experienced. Building on this framework, the quantitative analysis and assessment of policy outcomes could be advanced.

Through all this, just what is the nature of health and how does it compare with other benefits to be gained by economic activity? To begin with, is health improvement to be viewed as a private good, best left to the market, or is it a public good, calling for public intervention to overcome market failure? The answer depends on the particulars of the case and on how the problem is viewed. The individual patient, waiting for his pain pill to arrive, rightly views it as a private good, excludable and rival in consumption. Hence efficiency can be obtained in the market, and although government may enter to assure availability of medication as a matter of equity in distribution, it is not needed on efficiency grounds. The answer differs, however, when considering medication given to prevent the spread of communicable disease. With consumption now non-rival, the market fails in its provision and public financing is required.

Non-rival consumption may or may not be combined with excludability, and the role of the public hand differs accordingly. The advance of medical science, of medical 'knowing' of how to prevent and heal disease, is non-rival in use. Benefits to the consumer will be the larger, the more widely the given stock of knowledge is available, calling for its provision free of charge by the originator. This, however, would leave no compensation for those engaged in the advance of knowledge, and government must step in. Patent law might be used to preserve that incentive, limiting patent length so as to balance that gain against the immediate loss of not fully utilising the available stock of knowledge. Concern with the nature of public, private, and mixed goods thus provides an inseparable bond between health economics and public finance.

A further link between the two fields is provided by a shared concern with equity in distribution. In designing its budgets, the NHS applies two standards, choosing projects which are most effective in fighting particular diseases, and providing them in the most cost-efficient way. Alan agreed, but asserted that effectiveness and efficiency are not everything for 'behind them, there lurks equity'. Who should pay and who should benefit? How can health be measured, so that comparisons can be made and an equitable system be defined?

Fiscal equity, traditionally, has focused on the distribution of income across individuals, independent of its sources and uses. Severe inequality has been considered undesirable, with progressive taxation one of the correctives. But equity may also be viewed in 'categorical terms', and applied to the availability of goods which society views to be of particular importance (or 'merit goods' as they have come to be known). Among them, the availability of health services has been prominent. Publicly provided health services or support of privately provided services are used to correct for inequality in the patient's capacity to secure provision. Once more, there exists a link between fiscal and health economics.

Health services, like other goods, should be produced efficiently, and resources be spread across various diseases so as to maximise benefits at the margin; and personal care should be given to reduce the burden of illness. All this matters, but just who should benefit and who should pay? Equity enters throughout the health problem, across both its healing and care functions, but what is most needed is a formulation of the problem in manageable form. The ethical and philosophical issues, such as entitlement to equal health, the right to 'fair innings' and the right to live or die, must also be faced at the end, and this is where Alan's later work pointed. But the basics of measuring health, essential for the guidance of health policy, must be addressed first. Alan's choice to pursue health economics was indeed a perfect match for his humanity, good sense and talents, which have been the key to his path-breaking work.

CHAPTER 2

Citizens, consumers and clients: Alan Williams and the political economy of cost–benefit analysis

. . . Robert Sugden

INTRODUCTION

This paper focuses on the work of Alan Williams, the cost–benefit analyst, the predecessor of Alan Williams the leading health economist. In particular, it looks at Alan's involvement in early debates about the proper role of cost–benefit analysis (CBA) in the political process, about the relationships between the analyst, the agency commissioning a CBA and the wider community, and about the role of willingness-to-pay valuations in CBA. The issues that were involved in these debates remain relevant to current controversies about setting priorities in the delivery of health care – controversies that Alan continued to be engaged with until shortly before he died. The last time I met Alan – at a meeting in York in 2003 to discuss the methodology for a research project on 'the social value of a QALY' (quality-adjusted life year) – he was passionately defending a concept of 'social value' which can be traced back to the position he took in those early debates about CBA.

In trying to elucidate Alan's position, I will use two main texts. (I am going back to an era when academic economists published much less than they do now.) The first is the paper 'Cost–benefit analysis: bastard science? and/or insidious poison in the body politick?', which Alan wrote in 1970, and which was published in the first volume of *Journal of Public Economics* in 1972. The second is the book *The Principles of Practical Cost–benefit Analysis* which he and I wrote together over far too much of the 1970s, and which finally appeared in 1978 (Sugden and Williams, 1978). I will do my best to reconstruct from a fading memory the discussions through which we arrived at agreed positions, and in this way to separate Alan's views from mine.

COST–BENEFIT ANALYSIS AS MANAGEMENT CONSULTANCY: THE 'BASTARD SCIENCE?' PAPER

In striking contrast to the staid contents of more recent issues of *Journal of Public Economics*, Alan's paper (which from now on I will refer to as 'Bastard science?') begins with a satirical verse written in the style of WS Gilbert, entitled *The Management Consultant's Lament*. Alan reports that this verse was composed by a civil servant, JM Ross, as a response to Alan's 'own early activities' in the 'booming business of management consultancy' (Williams, 1972, p. 199). As this starting point suggests, Alan takes it as given that CBA *is a form of management consultancy*. His aim in the paper is to identify the features which distinguish CBA from other forms of consultancy, and to defend CBA against two charges: that it is a form of pseudoscience, and that, by substituting economic analysis for political deliberation and negotiation, it usurps democratic processes.

Alan starts from the premise that the objective of CBA is 'to assist choice[,] not to *make* choice'. He says that CBA is 'a natural and logical extension' of other techniques which serve the same purpose, such as systems analysis, operations research (OR) and cost-effectiveness analysis (Williams, 1972, pp. 200–201). Viewed in this perspective, CBA has two distinguishing features.

First, CBA is 'prescriptive'. Alan explains that, by this, he means that the analyst plays a 'consultative role'; the analysis is 'designed to help a client improve his situation' (p. 202). It is significant that the role of the analyst is defined in relation to that of a *client*: the client, presumably, is some agency (in the context of CBA, an agency of government) which is seeking assistance in making choices. The analyst's prescriptions take the form of advice about how the client agency can best achieve *its own* objective. This does not mean that the analyst's attitude towards the client has to be completely uncritical. Alan points out that clients often lack a clear sense of the nature of 'the problem' that they are asking the analyst to solve: 'any OR or CBA practitioner who accepts the client's initial formulation of the problem uncritically is heading for disaster' (Williams, 1972, p. 204). Still, it is clear that the analyst's role is to help the client to conceptualise *its* problem, as it perceives it, and not to prescribe what the client should be aiming to achieve.

The second, and most distinctive, feature of CBA is that it '[tries] hard to render inputs and outputs commensurable'. In its ideal form – an ideal that is not currently attainable – 'CBA will have all inputs and outputs evaluated in money terms' (Williams, 1972, pp. 200–202). However, Alan is at his most forceful in insisting that this does *not* mean that valuations should be based on individual willingness-to-pay.

Using Aaron Wildavsky as a spokesman for the claim that CBA is an insidious poison in the body politick, Alan quotes the following comment on CBA:

> The economic model on which cost–benefit analysis depends for its validity is based on a political theory. The idea is that in a free society the economy is to

> serve the individual's consistent preferences revealed and rationally pursued in the market place. Governments are not supposed to dictate preferences nor make decisions.
>
> (Wildavsky, 1966, p. 297)

Alan sees this as a gross misrepresentation: 'This is so patently false that if I had not had an opportunity to read and re-read this statement carefully I would not have believed it possible that such a well-informed and normally judicious observer could have made it' (Williams, 1972, p. 214). Alan accepts that 'much of the analysis that goes into most cost–benefit studies *is* based on the assumption that the market does constitute a good guide to the value of costs and benefits'; but he claims that the practice of CBA allows this assumption to be relaxed. Some of the relaxations he describes seem to me to be in the spirit of Wildavsky's account of CBA. For example, Alan says that CBA 'may require . . . valuations inferred from market behaviour to be placed on items which have no market values'; but this is a case in which the government is *eliciting* preferences, not *dictating* them. Alan's crucial objection is that CBA 'may require . . . the use of valuations postulated by the policy-makers or decision-makers themselves' (Williams, 1972, p. 214).

The legitimacy of such *postulated values* is a recurring theme in the paper. For example, he accepts that if 'a client (say a Minister of Transport) [says] that for the purposes of this analysis I want variable *X* valued at £*Y* per unit (where *X* might be the intrinsic value of life)', then '£*Y* represents a precise statement about the client's policy trade-off between *X* and the other variables in the analysis', and so is a legitimate datum for CBA. This kind of postulated value is 'arbitrary' in the sense that it is not supported by evidence, but it is not 'irresponsible' because 'it does imply a commitment to allocate resources in a particular way for which the client will have to answer', and 'it provides a precise focus for discussion by others (say Cabinet colleagues) who might wish to influence his judgements on this matter or modify their own' (Williams, 1972, p. 210). Notice that, in this account, postulated values are presented as internal to the government machine. There is no suggestion of public debate about these values, apart from the hint that the government may ultimately have to answer to its electorate.

Here is how Alan sums up his position on the status of market-based and postulated values in CBA:

> I am doing no more than accepting the well-recognised proposition that you cannot ascribe values without making value judgements. Market prices are acceptable if the value-premises underlying market behaviour are acceptable (e.g. accepting the prevailing distribution of economic power and the relevance of individual market-oriented valuations to the making of social judgements) . . . Postulated prices are acceptable if it is believed that the value-premises

> underlying both market and imputed prices are misconceived for the purpose in hand (e.g. if one accepts the propriety of a paternalistic or collectivist basis for valuation).
>
> (Williams, 1972, p. 220)

The reader is entitled to ask: *Who* is making the value judgements here? *To whom* are postulated prices acceptable or unacceptable? The logic of the paper as a whole seems to allow only one answer: the client.

Summing up: Alan's position in 'Bastard science?' is that CBA is a particularly ambitious form of management consultancy. It is scientific in the sense of being systematic: 'assumptions are required to be explicit, evidence presented, results communicable and replicable' (Williams, 1972, p. 203). It does not usurp the political process because it does not claim to make decisions and does not impose any substantive value judgements; it merely assists clients to formulate their own objectives and to pursue them effectively.

TWO OPPOSING VIEWS OF COST–BENEFIT ANALYSIS: THE PRINCIPLES OF PRACTICAL COST–BENEFIT ANALYSIS

Before discussing the text of *The Principles of Practical Cost–benefit Analysis* (Sugden and Williams, 1978), I need to explain how the book came to be written, and Alan's and my respective roles as co-authors.

My becoming an economist was very largely due to Alan. I was an undergraduate at York between 1967 and 1970, studying history and economics. The topic in economics that most interested me was CBA, which I learned about from Alan's lecture course on investment appraisal. For my final-year project, I chose to do a retrospective cost–benefit study of the recent closure of the Whitby–Scarborough railway. Alan was my supervisor, and went far beyond the requirements of duty in helping me to make contact with various agencies that were able to provide me with data I needed. He had gently suggested to me that the plan of carrying out a complete cost–benefit study was over-ambitious for one student over a summer vacation, but I wanted to (and, I think, did) prove him wrong. While reading the reports of previous cost–benefit studies of rail closures, I had my first genuinely original economic idea: I realised that the methodology that had been used by the Ministry of Transport in its most recent rail-closure study made a theoretical error in its treatment of changes in fare revenue. When I told Alan that I had discovered this error, I sensed that he was sceptical, but he listened to my argument in his characteristically open-minded way. After some thought, he agreed that I was right. He encouraged me to write a paper on the subject and send it to the *Bulletin of Economic Research*; this became my first publication (Sugden, 1972). The following summer, I had my first paid job as an economist, working for Alan on a project he had persuaded the University of York to finance, investigating whether the apparent scarcity of private-sector student accommodation in the city could be reduced by making suitable adjustments to bus routes. (This is a good illustration of Alan's conception of the creative role of the analyst. The university perceived its problem as a shortage of student accommodation in areas accessible to the campus; Alan saw that the problem could be restated as the poor accessibility of otherwise suitable areas).

After a year studying for a master's degree in Cardiff, I returned to York in 1971, as by far the economics department's youngest and least-qualified lecturer. Shortly after this, Oxford University Press invited Alan to write a textbook on CBA. He had a very clear idea about the kind of book that was needed – an idea expressed in the apparently paradoxical title he chose for it. It should be *practical* in orientation, teaching would-be analysts how to provide useful advice to clients, using simplified case studies as a method of instruction and as training exercises. But it should not be a cookbook, presenting CBA as a set of techniques to be applied mechanically; it should induct its readers into the general *principles* on which CBA was based. In fact, it should follow the strategy of his investment appraisal lecture course. Since he didn't have time to write this much-needed book on his own, he suggested that we took on the project as co-authors – I doing most of the actual writing, but under his general guidance and, of course, with his reputation to sell the book. (I should say that he insisted that almost all the royalties came to me.)

In many ways, *The Principles of Practical Cost–benefit Analysis* was, for me, the equivalent of writing a PhD thesis (something I never did); Alan's role was similar to that of a thesis supervisor, except that the final text had to be in a form that he could sign up to. At first, I didn't expect this to be much of a problem. However, just as PhD supervisees usually do, I gradually developed a perspective of my own, and it became more difficult for us to reach agreement on what our book should say. Increasingly, I felt the pull of currents of thought in economics which ran counter to Alan's understanding of CBA.

In the early 1970s, economists' views about the nature of CBA began to polarise. One school of thought was essentially that of 'Bastard science?'. On this view, CBA is a branch of economic planning; the key ideas it imports from economics are those of optimisation theory. There are no *a priori* restrictions on the objective function to be maximised. This position was taken by Ian Little and James Mirrlees in their influential text, *Project Appraisal and Planning for Developing Countries* (1974). However, there was an opposing school of thought, represented by Ezra Mishan's equally influential *Cost–benefit Analysis* (1971). On this view, CBA is the applied branch of what in 1971 was still 'new' welfare economics – that is, the welfare economics of the Kaldor–Hicks compensation test. The key ideas that CBA imports from economics are those of welfare economics, consumer theory and price theory, particularly the concepts of producers' and consumers' surplus. The task of the cost–benefit analyst is to investigate whether the total amount that those who would gain from a policy proposal would be willing to pay for their gains is greater or less than the total amount that losers would be willing to accept as compensation. On this account, the cost–benefit analyst is an independent specialist, committed to applying a particular set of evaluative principles. A client who employs such a specialist cannot ask for those principles to be changed: he pays to be told what they imply in a specific case. There is simply no place in CBA for postulated values. Mishan, I think, would have endorsed the quotation from Wildavsky (*see* pp. 6–7) which Alan thought patently false.

Another pull came from the theory of public choice, one of the intellectual growth areas of the 1970s and part of the wave of 'New Right' thinking which paved the way for Margaret Thatcher's election victory in 1979. A central theme of public choice theory was the implausibility of (what was then) the conventional economist's view of government as a benevolent despot or *deus ex machina*, a neutral force which could be called in to correct market failures. The public choice literature taught economists to see political failure as just as much a problem as market failure, and to model the behaviour of government agencies in terms of the interactions of individually motivated actors. Alan's conception of the 'client' for CBA began to sound suspiciously like the non-existent benevolent despot.

Also built in to much of the theory of public choice was the hypothesis that when individuals act as voters and when they act in the market, they are acting on the same preferences: at the level of the individual, there is no distinction between the 'citizen' and the 'consumer'. (Let me say in passing that I am no longer persuaded of the truth of this hypothesis.) Anyone who accepts this hypothesis will have difficulty with Alan's idea that one might conclude that 'the value-premises underlying both market and imputed prices are misconceived for the purpose in hand' and that one might instead accept 'the propriety of a paternalistic or collectivist basis for valuation' (Williams, 1972, p. 220). The value-premises underlying market prices, one would have to conclude, are simply the preferences of the individuals who act in the market. As voters, those same individuals have the same preferences. So when a government agency declares that these value-premises are misconceived, it is declaring that it is choosing not to act in accordance with the preferences of the people who elect it and pay for it. How can this be justified *to those people*?

In responding to these currents of thought, I was influenced by other York colleagues, particularly Mike Jones-Lee and Tony Culyer, and later by James Buchanan. Mike Jones-Lee was a firm adherent of Mishan's approach to CBA. His pioneering work on eliciting ordinary individuals' valuations of reductions in risks of premature death was showing that it was possible to construct willingness-to-pay valuations even of 'statistical life' (Jones-Lee, 1976); he convinced me that this was a better way for CBA to deal with risks of death than the use of postulated values. More generally, the analysis of individual willingness to pay was in the spirit of the York department's tradition of applied microeconomics. At the time, Tony Culyer was producing imaginative analyses of real-world problems using only the simple components of Marshallian price theory, with a touch of populist scepticism about governments which increasingly appealed to me. I had the good fortune to be able to spend the summer of 1977 at Buchanan's Public Choice Centre in Blacksburg, Virginia, and felt an immediate attraction to his contractarian form of normative economics, in which the role of government is not to judge what is good for society, but to implement projects which individuals recognise as being in their mutual interest. This was just after Alan and I had finished our book, but the ideas which crystallised for me in Blacksburg had been forming long before that.

So how did Alan and I manage to complete our book? Despite the famous placard on his desk, Alan's line was never 'Be reasonable: do it my way'. Rather, he looked for ways in which we could acknowledge our fundamental differences within the structure of a practically oriented textbook. The original plan of the book, as designed by Alan, served us well. As in 'Bastard science?', we conceptualised the appraisal process as a dialogue between 'the analyst' and 'the decision maker' (Alan's 'client'). In order for analysis to be possible, we said, the decision maker's objective needed to be specified. The kind of analysis that was required depended on the nature of that objective. In many contexts, even in the public sector, agencies are expected to act on 'commercial criteria' – that is, to use financial appraisal. So we began by explaining the principles of financial appraisal. This relatively uncontroversial material took up the first third of the book.

We then suggested that public decision makers might be expected to take account of a wider range of policy effects than can be encompassed by financial appraisal. As one way of doing this, we introduced the compensation test. At this point, we distinguished between two ways of thinking about CBA – the *decision-making approach* (Alan's preferred approach, in which the objective is whatever the decision maker chooses it to be) and the *Paretian approach* (Mishan's approach, in which CBA is seen as an application of Paretian welfare economics, and the objective is given by the compensation test). However, we began by playing down this distinction, presenting the compensation criterion as a simple and tractable way of taking account of a wide range of effects in a consistent way; as such, it provides a credible 'first approximation to a full statement of government objectives', even within the decision-making approach (Sugden and Williams, 1978, p. 93). This kept us going for another third of the book, in which we dealt with shadow pricing, consumers' and producers' surplus, imputed prices and uncertainty. It was only in the final third of the book that we introduced the idea of postulated values – for particular goods such as health care, for weighting gains and losses to different income groups, and in the form of a postulated social discount rate. Here, things became more awkward as we repeatedly reminded the reader that the legitimacy of postulated values was a controversial issue, and tried to treat the two approaches to CBA even-handedly.

In the final chapter, entitled 'Epilogue: the analyst, the decision-maker and the community', we reworked some of the themes of 'Bastard science?', with the significant difference that the analyst and decision maker were placed in a triangular relationship with 'the community as a whole'. We declared that 'the public decision-maker is entrusted to act on behalf of this community' (Sugden and Williams, 1978, pp. 220–30). Clearly, the intention was to qualify Alan's earlier account of CBA as management consultancy, by making both analyst and client responsible to a wider community. My recollection is that the idea that we should do this was originally mine, but that Alan worked over my drafts quite closely, suggesting revisions and making sure that he could endorse the sentiments expressed.

The idea that the analyst has responsibilities beyond those of a consultant to a client was developed in two ways. The first (which, as far as I can recall, Alan supported wholeheartedly), appeals to a professional ethic of intellectual honesty. In the perspective of the decision-making approach, one of the principal virtues of CBA is *consistency*. It is by making different decisions of the same agency consistent with one another, and consistent with a common objective, that CBA promotes efficiency in the allocation of resources. However, if the benefits of efficiency are to be achieved, the CBA must be done in good faith and not as mere window-dressing. The more freedom decision makers have to specify their own objectives and to postulate their own values, the more scope there is for self-serving window-dressing. I think I felt at the time – and I certainly believe now – that this is a serious weakness of the decision-making approach. The less discretion there is for CBA methodology to be tailored to specific appraisals, or even to the interests of specific commissioning agencies or governments, the more confidence one can have that the results are genuinely informative. On these grounds, I now favour the convention that CBA should be based on individual willingness to pay (*see* Sugden, 2005). But back in the mid-1970s, I was still making up my mind. Alan and I were able to sign up to the claim that, if consistency is a virtue of CBA, the analyst's professional role must include the advocacy of consistency, even in cases in which the client would prefer to be inconsistent. Thus, in reporting the results of a cost–benefit study, the analyst has a professional responsibility to point out the wider implications of using whatever values have been postulated for that study (Sugden and Williams, 1978, pp. 231–6).

The second form of responsibility is to the community as a whole. My recollection is that we had more difficulty agreeing on the passages which deal with this issue. We discussed it in relation to another virtue of CBA, *explicitness*. We pointed out that the explicitness of CBA is not always desired by clients: their interests may sometimes be better served by obfuscation. However (and here the influence of public choice theory can be detected), explicitness might have a corresponding value to the community as a whole, as a mechanism of accountability:

> Thus cost–benefit analysis should not be seen solely as a service to the decision-maker. If the analysis is not secret, it exposes the logic of the decision-maker's

> actions to the scrutiny of those to whom he is accountable . . . [It] carries a stage further the function of traditional financial accounting. The obligation on the part of privately owned firms and public agencies to keep financial accounts is a very effective deterrent against embezzlement and fraud by managers, public officials and politicians. The obligation to justify public decisions within the framework of cost–benefit analysis discourages a much subtler form of abuse of responsibility – that of taking decisions on behalf of others by using criteria that these others would not approve.
>
> (Sugden and Williams, 1978, p. 240)

Significantly, our concept of accountability allowed political decision makers to choose objectives and postulate values. We offered the following understanding of the political process (cautiously prefaced by 'one can argue that'):

> the role of the analyst is to assist, not simply a decision-maker, but a decision-making process that has the assent of the community as a whole . . . The decision-maker is responsible for making a decision, according to his own lights, but he is responsible to the community. His right to decide stems from the consent of the community, expressed through the political system. The community, then, ought to have the right to call upon the decision-maker to account for his decisions.
>
> (Sugden and Williams, 1978, p. 241)

This formulation leaves room for CBA to be based on the kind of 'collectivist' value premises that featured in 'Bastard science?'. The claim that these premises are *social* values is still only a value judgement made by the decision maker *on behalf of* the community: there is no requirement that this judgement is endorsed by the members of the community themselves. But there is a recognition that the decision maker has to account for his judgements to the people on whose behalf he claims to make them.

CITIZENS AND CONSUMERS IN ALAN WILLIAMS' HEALTH ECONOMICS

The views expressed in the Epilogue of *The Principles of Practical Cost–benefit Analysis* (Sugden and Williams, 1978) seem to occupy an intermediate position between the 'Bastard science?' account of CBA as management consultancy and the conception of the role of the health economist that is implicit in Alan's later work.

On my (far from complete) reading of Alan's work in health economics, his central research programme *was* a form of CBA, in the main senses in which he defined CBA in 'Bastard science?'. It was prescriptive, designed to assist choices about the allocation of resources within publicly financed healthcare systems. And it was committed to the aim of making inputs and outputs as commensurable as possible. The whole point of the QALY, for which he was such a dedicated advocate, was to try to make the outputs of the healthcare industry commensurable with one another. Alan was always clear-sighted in recognising that priority setting was an inescapable part of medical decision making, and that allocative efficiency implied a shadow-price for a QALY (or shadow-prices for QALYs accruing to different classes of beneficiary). However, he never accepted that QALYs should be valued in terms of willingness to pay. (This was what was at dispute in the meeting in 2003, which I mentioned in the introduction. In a reprise of the York of the 1970s, but with some interesting re-alignments of ideological positions, Mike Jones-Lee and I argued for the willingness-to-pay approach, while Tony Culyer inclined to Alan's position.) In this sense, Alan maintained his commitment to the legitimacy of postulated values.

However, Alan's conception of the 'client' – the audience to which his work was addressed, and the source of postulated values – seems to have undergone some change. He sought to engage, not only with public decision makers, but also with the wider community of people who use public health services and who pay for them through their taxes. Crucially, he sought to engage with them as citizens and not as consumers.

In a paper of 1988, with the title 'Priority setting in public and private health care: a guide through the ideological jungle', Alan nails his own colours to the mast. He argues that, despite the messy mix of public and private elements that we find in all real healthcare systems, there is a fundamental ideological divide between 'libertarian' and 'egalitarian' viewpoints about the provision of health care. In a libertarian healthcare system, the 'dominant ethic' is 'willingness and ability to pay', while in an egalitarian system, it is 'equal opportunity of access for those in equal need' (Williams, 1988, p. 174). Alan asks us to commit ourselves to one ethic or the other: 'Each of us must decide for ourselves where we stand in that particular configuration of attitudes, and be honest with ourselves and with others about it'. He declares himself an egalitarian. Although these commitments are made by us as individual citizens, Alan argues that what is ultimately required is a *collective* decision about which of the two ideological positions is to govern the provision of health care in a given political community.

He rejects the suggestion that there can be a mixed solution, of the kind that a contractarian might favour, in which there is a socialised system of health care for those who value social insurance and are prepared to pay for it collectively, and a market-based system for those who choose to opt out and provide for themselves:

> I feel quite strongly egalitarian, and would aim to make the public system stronger and the private system weaker, in any community on which I depend for health care. But I also recognise the need, in a democratic country, to

> respect the ideological position of the minority, provided it is not actually subversive. The trouble with private systems, in my view, is that they become 'subversive' if permitted to play a *significant* role in a mixed system, because public systems rely on strong feelings of social solidarity (the rich must help the poor, the healthy the sick, the wise the foolish, the well-informed the ignorant, and so on), whereas private systems exist precisely to enable the rich, healthy, wise and well-informed to 'opt out' and look after themselves.
>
> (Williams, 1988, p. 182)

The implication is that a fundamental collective decision has to be made about which set of values is to predominate. When it comes to the setting of priorities, each type of healthcare system 'has to be judged according to its own lights, i.e. according to its own ideology' (Williams, 1988, p. 183). In his work as a health economist, Alan starts from the premise that, in the UK, a collective decision has already been made in favour of the use of egalitarian values. This prior decision sets the ground rules for political debate about healthcare priorities.

Thus, in a discussion piece on age-based rationing, published in the *British Medical Journal* (*BMJ*) in 1997, Alan poses the question: Whose values should count in a social insurance setting? He asks us to suppose that older people are willing to pay more than younger people for health improvements for themselves. Is that relevant for the setting of priorities in the NHS? Alan insists it is not:

> But did we not take the NHS out of that [private market] context precisely because as citizens (rather than as consumers of health care) we were pursuing a rather different ideal – namely, that health care should be provided according to people's needs, not according to what they were each willing and able to pay[?] A person's needs (constituting claims on social resources) have to be arbitrated by a third party, whose unenviable task it is to weigh different needs (and different people's needs) one against another. This is precisely what priority setting in health care is all about. So the values of the citizenry as a whole must override the values of a particular interest group within it.
>
> (Williams, 1997a)

So, Alan is declaring, the setting of healthcare priorities in the NHS must be based on judgements about relative need, made by a 'third party'. The reference to the 'unenviable task' strongly suggests that the third party is a political or professional decision maker – someone like the 'client' of 'Bastard science?' or the 'decision-maker' of *Principles of Practical Cost–benefit Analysis*. The implication seems to be that priorities are set *by* the decision-maker, *on behalf of* 'the citizenry as a whole'.

Much more than in his earlier work on CBA, however, Alan the health economist wants to draw the citizenry into the priority-setting process. A major part of Alan's research programme in health economics has been concerned with eliciting, from representative samples of the population, citizen-perspective judgements about marginal trade-offs between different healthcare benefits and different classes of beneficiary. In the *BMJ* paper, he appeals to evidence from surveys which show that most people, including the old themselves, favour giving priority to the health care of the young (*see* also Williams, 1997b, p. 118). The implication is that this is relevant evidence for decision makers. In addition, Alan clearly wanted to foster public debate about priorities. Thus, in the *BMJ* paper, he offers the hope that 'reasonable limits' on the demands for health care that the old can make on their fellow citizens can be set 'with fairly general consent', and (as an elderly man) he appeals to the members of his generation to exercise restraint in the political demands they make on the healthcare system.

As an example of Alan's conception of the relationship between the decision maker and the community, consider the following passage. He is responding to an argument by Amartya Sen that the principle of non-discrimination between the sexes in the delivery of health care should take priority over the pursuit of equality in lifetime health experience. (Since men have shorter life expectancy than women, equalising access to QALYs between the sexes would require discrimination in favour of men.) Alan notes that, following Sen, one might draw up a list of 'possible axes of discrimination' and make *a priori* moral judgements about the acceptability or unacceptability of discrimination on each axis:

> But this is not the path I would take. I would prefer to find out from people generally at what point they would be willing to discriminate (and how strongly) when told the amount of damage such a moral constraint is causing to the important aim of reducing inequalities in lifetime experience in health . . . I would then compare the median trade-off rate from my representative sample of the population with the shadow price of the restriction as it currently operates, and then decide, in the light of the results, whether to accept the status quo or start thinking of ways of tightening up or relaxing the moral constraint.
>
> (Williams, 2003, p. 65)

I take it that, by 'the path I would take', Alan means the path that he would take *as a public decision maker*, charged with setting healthcare priorities. He is disagreeing with Sen on two levels. As a good economist, he is rejecting the idea of absolute moral constraints in favour of marginal trade-offs between different objectives. But he is also rejecting the idea that public decisions should be governed by the moral principles that decision makers (or moral philosophers) deem to be good or right. Instead, he proposes to investigate the judgements that are in fact made by informed citizens. Notice that his survey respondents are not being asked to compare different combinations of healthcare benefits and costs *for themselves*; they are being asked to play the role of third-party arbitrator. Notice also that Alan's decision maker appears to be reserving to himself the final decision about what to do 'in the light of the results'. It seems that the survey of citizen judgements is intended to *inform* that decision, not to *make* it.

There is, I suggest, an essential continuity from the account of CBA in 'Bastard science?', through the 'decision-making approach' of *The Principles of Practical Cost–benefit Analysis*, to Alan's approach to health economics. Throughout, Alan has been committed to a conception of political decision-making in which policy options are assessed in relation to an objective which in some way expresses a collective judgement of the relevant community. His inclination, I think, has always been to see applied microeconomics as addressed to an imagined public decision maker who is ultimately responsible for deciding, on behalf of the community, what the collective objective is to be. He has consistently rejected the idea that this objective can be constructed from the preferences that individuals reveal as consumers, whether in the market or in response to questions about their willingness to pay for private benefits. However, and particularly in his later work, he has expected public decision makers to be responsive to the judgements that individuals make as informed citizens. My contractarian leanings prevent me from endorsing this approach; but no one can do more than Alan to make it reasonable.

ACKNOWLEDGEMENTS

My work on this paper was supported by the Economic and Social Research Council (award no RES 051 27 0146).

REFERENCES

Jones-Lee M (1976) *The Value of Life: an economic analysis*. London: Martin Robertson and Chicago University Press.

Little I and Mirrlees J (1974) *Project Appraisal and Planning for Developing Countries*. London: Heinemann Educational.

Mishan E (1971) *Cost–benefit Analysis*. London: Allen and Unwin.

Sugden R (1972) Cost–benefit analysis and the withdrawal of railway services. *Bulletin of Economic Research* **24**: 23–32.

Sugden R (2005) Coping with preference anomalies in cost–benefit analysis: a market-simulation approach. *Environmental and Resource Economics* **32**: 129–60.

Sugden R and Williams A (1978) *The Principles of Practical Cost–benefit Analysis*. New York, Oxford: Oxford University Press.

Wildavsky A (1966) The political economy of efficiency: cost–benefit analysis, systems analysis and program budgeting. *Public Administration Review* **26**: 292–310.

Williams A (1972) Cost–benefit analysis: bastard science? and/or insidious poison in the body politick? *Journal of Public Economics* **1**: 199–225.

Williams A (1988) Priority setting in public and private health care: a guide through the ideological jungle. *Journal of Health Economics* **7**: 173–83.

Williams A (1997a) The rationing debate: rationing health care by age: the case for. *British Medical Journal* **314**: 820.

Williams A (1997b) Intergenerational equity: an exploration of the 'fair innings' argument. *Health Economics* **6**: 117–32.

Williams A (2003) Comment on Amartya Sen's 'Why health equity'. *Health Economics* **12**: 65–6.

CHAPTER 3

Alan Williams and cost–benefit analysis in health care: comments on the paper by Robert Sugden

. . . Bengt Jönsson

INTRODUCTION

For me, Alan Williams the cost–benefit analyst is synonymous with Alan Williams the leading health economist. His major research was on the methods and application of economic evaluations to resource allocation in health care.

Bob Sugden (BS) rightly points out that Williams' 1972 paper was inspired by the shift of interest in public economics from public finance to public expenditure analysis, and particularly PPB (planning, programme, budgeting) analysis, that occurred in the 1960s, and which drew critique from political scientists like Wildavsky (Wildavsky, 1973). Economists thus come into a role as 'management consultants' to governments, to help improve the use of the resources raised from taxation, thus competing with the political scientists as advisors. To meet the critic there was a need to define the criteria for what was included, and not included, in a cost–benefit analysis.

Alan Williams' (hereafter known affectionately as 'AW') 'Bastard science?' paper triggered my first visit to York. Although I approached him as a 'cost–benefit' analyst, he introduced me to the concept of 'health economics' (Cooper and Culyer, 1973), and the visit prompted a shift in my research interest towards application of CBA in health. The idea for my planned PhD thesis was very close to Alan's idea for the textbook that he was invited to write at about the same time: to review the published studies in the field with the objective of systematising and comparing, and to find a possible common theoretical base (principles). It should not be yet another 'bad example' of an applied study without a clear method, nor a cookbook of how to perform studies. The aim was to reveal and develop the practices and principles involved. The work on my dissertation, which benefited very much from continued contacts with AW and members of the Health Economics Working Group (HEWG) during that time, was thus parallel to AW's and BS's work with the textbook to be published in 1978 (Sugden and Williams, 1978).

When the dissertation was completed and ready to be defended, the faculty chose AW to act as opponent (Jönsson, 1976). The defence of the dissertation is an important academic institution in Swedish academic life, where a leading researcher in the field is asked by the faculty to review and critique the thesis in public. It is not so common that the opponent is asked to document his 'opposition', but AW's comments were considered so 'helpful and enlightening' (quote from preface by Lars Söderström, Head, Department of Economics, Lund University) that he was asked to include his notes in the department's series of seminar papers (Williams, 1976). Since his comments probably are not much known outside Lund, I will quote them extensively to contrast, or rather reinforce the observations BS makes in his paper. I will raise the following questions for discussion:

1 what was AW's position on CBA in general and in its application to health in particular?
2 how can it be explained, what was the rationale?
3 what were the implications and consequences of his position?

ALAN WILLIAMS' POSITION ON CBA

I have no objections to BS's description of AW's position, which I would like to summarise as follows:

The role of CBA in the decision-making process

- Should be scientific, yet practical and based on explicit values
- Should be aimed at helping decision makers do better.

Critique of Paretian welfare economics

- Based on willingness to pay (WTP) and ability to pay which is rejected as a resource allocation principle in health care
- The decision-maker approach (management consultancy?) is an alternative.

The methodology of CBA

- Market-based values and willingness to pay is only acceptable for valuation of resources (the cost side)
- Postulated values for health benefits based on decision-maker values
- Developed into cost per QALY as a general method for the application of CBA to health.

His position could be contrasted to the essential positions taken in my dissertation:

- acceptance of a public healthcare system where everybody has access to health care, but where few, if any, decision makers care about efficiency in resource allocation
- CBA is needed, particularly for decisions about new technology, but practice must be improved – studies are not comparable
- there is *government failure* as well as *market failure*, and CBA is a method to correct both
- welfare economics should guide application and method for CBA
- the value of health improvements should be assessed through expressed WTP from a citizen perspective (insurance method).

Alan started his opposition with the statement: 'I see my role as being that of bringing to Bengt Jönsson's work the perspective of a non-Scandinavian observer of the cost–benefit scene, who has recently devoted a large part of his time to the planning and evaluation of health services (especially in Britain) with the object of exploring the potential of the tools and insights of economics'. AW's views on CBA were formed by his attempts to apply economics to the healthcare sector. For me, AW the CBA analyst and AW the health economist are very much the same thing. He had formed his position over a number of years, as evident from the four papers he is referring to in the notes for his opposition (Williams, 1974a–c, 1977). His views expressed in his comments on the thesis reflect his position in the middle of the work on his book together with BS.

AW was very determined in the view that the role of CBA is to assist decisions, not to make them (the insidious poison critique). While I subscribed to the same view 'The purpose of the thesis is to demonstrate "the way in which economic theory and method can be used to clarify the resource problems in the medical sector, to assist choice not to make choice"' (AW quoting from the dissertation). However, I have a feeling that he was not totally satisfied with the word 'clarify' in my statement. Even if the 'management consultant' is not the responsible decision maker, his role is to help the decision maker to arrive at a conclusion, given his objectives and the constraints. To limit the role of the economist to investigate whether a particular resource allocation was efficient according to the Kaldor–Hicks criteria, which was the position I explored in the thesis, was not in his mind, as we will see later.

WHAT IS THE ECONOMIST'S PARTICULAR CONTRIBUTION?

AW stressed the need for a *clearly* defined decision problem. The role of the health economist, in his role as management consultant, was to help the decision maker to define the problem. He stressed that it is 'hardly ever a decision about "ALL OR NOTHING"' and he continued 'of all the major themes in the study, this is probably the most important contribution of economists to problem formulation (and why it is so silly to regard them simply as hirelings to be brought in after the real work has been done, to add a touch of cosmetic costing to an ill-designed study)' (Williams, 1976).

Another role for the economist is to 'make sure *all* relevant costs/benefits are included, but only once'. Thus AW subscribed to social cost perspective and not a specific decision-maker perspective. He noted that 'CBA is not the same as financial appraisal', it should have a 'GNP [gross national product] orientation (opportunity cost of time)' and that also resources 'not in GDP [gross domestic product] (time lost for persons not in the labour force)' should be included (Williams, 1976).

In a later paper (Williams, 1981) he develops this, stating that 'When we assume that all changes in real resources associated with the alternative under investigation have been measured, it is useful to classify them as:

a. changes in resources used in service production
b. changes in resources used by patients and their helpers
c. changes in gross domestic product'.

While he also stated that 'the benefit measure shall not depend on the wealth or "economic" value of the individual', he never addressed the problem that benefits/costs should be included 'only once'. It may, for example be difficult to measure health improvements as the number of QALYs gained, without differences in resources (costs and income) between states not affecting the estimate. See for example the discussion about to what extent indirect costs are included in measures of the utility of a health state (Gold *et al.*, 1996).

THE PURPOSE OF COST–BENEFIT ANALYSIS, AND ALAN WILLIAMS' CRITIQUE OF PARETIAN WELFARE ECONOMICS

AW subscribed to the view that the role of CBA was to assist administrative decisions, not clinical ones. However, he pointed out that clinical freedom was restricted by resource constraints, which meant that we have to move beyond the medical ethic 'to do good, and no harm', to make decisions about where extra resources produced the greatest health benefit (a social and citizen perspective).

AW agreed with me that both market failure and distributional goals constitute a need for CBA. But he had some qualification regarding the distributional goals, and added a merit goods argument ('assessment of need') that was not in the thesis; i.e. 'paternalism' rather than 'consumerism'. 'Whether this is as it should be or not is a lively and controversial area of debate into which I will not enter at present. *But* if it is conceded *that as a matter of fact* it is quite a common phenomenon, then we have to ask whether the economist's role is thereby emasculated (which I suspect is Jönsson's position) or whether we should press on and try to systematise what will otherwise tend to be an obscure area of unanalysed mystique (which is my preferred strategy, of which more later)' (Williams, 1976).

While I advocated assessments of WTP for health improvements *before* illness strikes (insurance method) (Jönsson, 1977) to overcome the ability to pay objection, he was not totally convinced. 'This [unequal income distribution in relation to need] can be overcome by experiments designed to elicit relative valuations in contexts in which purchasing power is constant, but it may be better to resort to "proxy" valuers, via the political process, or even to rely on "experts", provided their values are brought into the open'. And he continues '. . . it may well be more efficient to delegate the decision to people who know more about it, even if they *are* imperfect judges of consumers' valuations', and '. . . Even if they *were* "well-informed", patients may not be the best judges of their own welfare' (Williams, 1976).

I interpreted consumers here to be citizens/the general population. Perhaps that is a mistake, and AW instead meant 'patients'. If that is the case, he is consistent with his later position not to use valuations of patients in the actual health states for valuation of the utility to be in those states.

AW ON THE WAY FORWARD

Alternatives to Paretian Welfare Economics

> There is an alternative view, which I espouse, which is that the economist's contribution to CBA is not restricted by the confines of Paretian Welfare Economics, but that, since we have special skills and expertise in handling valuation problems, we can (and should) go boldly into the territory of the valuation of 'need' by practitioners and policy makers as well as analysing compensation awards by judges and any other sources of information on 'social' values (Williams, 1976).

> Systematic studies of practitioners and the concepts of health they use as well as the relative weights (valuations) they attach to the various dimensions of health. Work with medical researchers in the development of *health status indexes* (Williams, 1976).

Valuation of healthiness *per se*:

> This work is *not* constrained within the Paretian straitjacket, but nor is it *mystical* and *obscurantist* and beyond analysis, for it has its own clear conceptual basis and rigorous measurement criteria (Williams, 1976).

And some advice to a PhD student:

> I would hope to persuade thoughtful scholars like Bengt Jönsson that the pure Paretian doctrine, à la Mishan, has outlived its usefulness, and is now merely a

starting point for work in this field, and one which we can safely move beyond in the field of health economics (Williams, 1976).

IMPLICATIONS AND CONSEQUENCES OF HIS POSITION

AW understood early on that CBA is a valuable tool for improving resource allocation in health care, and he was very effective in communicating this insight. He stressed that CBA can and should be based on good science, and that CBA should 'clarify' the resource allocation problem, not make the decision. He did not take very great interest in discussing costs, but from what he wrote he took the position that CBA should be based on a social cost concept, and that distributional aspects should be addressed. The development of the QALY as an outcome measure was a major step forward in the practical application of economic evaluation in health care.

His critique of Paretian welfare economics as a theoretical base for CBA was very strong and effective, because it came from someone with deep knowledge about the subject. A consequence of this was that very few young health economists were brave enough to explore the opportunities of developing the WTP approach to valuation of health improvements. However, I interpret his objections based as much on practice as on principles. Welfare economics was used for formulating arguments against public health care, particularly in the US, and he was a firm defender of a public healthcare system. For a health economist coming from a country were there was unanimous support for an egalitarian publicly funded healthcare system, this was not a major issue. However, it is understandable if AW looked at it differently, since the NHS was founded in 1948 and was therefore less established than, for example, the public healthcare systems in the Nordic countries. Another important aspect, which AW probably sensed before other economists, was that WTP and the monetary valuation of health were rejected by decision makers, clinicians as well as administrators and politicians, in most healthcare systems in Europe, and probably also the US. My conclusion is that AW made a careful evaluation of what was needed for health economics to be accepted within the healthcare system. Even if WTP estimates could be adjusted to meet equity criteria, they may have been rejected by decisions makers.* For AW it was more important to improve practice than to be right in principle.

It also turned out that he advocated, and over 30 years developed, the right principles to be practical, making an outstanding contribution to making CBA a scientific method and an accepted and useful tool for improving health policy. AW did not need any 'Paretian straitjacket', but I think I share the conviction with BS that it is useful to have this available for CBA management consultants who do not have the integrity and intellectual standing of AW.

* Note the difference with CBA within environmental economics, where WTP is the gold standard, and where this method is much more developed.

Working closely with decision makers to help them to make decisions about the allocation of healthcare resources in the public interest is an important, but also a challenging, role. AW is a great example of how it can be done, and a role model for many of us who have tried.

REFERENCES

Cooper M and AJ Culyer (eds) (1973) *Health Economics: selected readings.* Harmondsworth: Penguin.

Gold MR, Siegel JE, Russell LB and Weinstein MC (1996) *Cost-effectiveness in Health and Medicine.* New York: Oxford University Press.

Jönsson B (1976) *Cost–benefit Analysis in Public Health and Medical Care* [dissertation] Lund University: Department of Economics.

Jönsson B (1977) Application of cost benefit analysis to health problems In: Halberstadt V and Culyer AJ (eds) *Public Economics and Human Resources.* Proceeding of the 31st Congress of the International Institute of Public Finance. Paris: Editions Cujas, pp. 193–202.

Sugden R and Williams A (1978) *The Principles of Practical Cost-benefit Analysis.* Oxford: Oxford University Press.

Wildavsky A (1973) If planning is everything, maybe it's nothing. *Policy Sciences* **4**: 127–53.

Williams A (1974a) Measuring the effectiveness of health care systems. *British Journal of Preventive and Social Medicine* **28**: 196–202.

Williams A (1974b) Need as a demand concept (with special reference to health). In: Culyer AJ (ed.) *Economic Policies and Social Goals.* London: Martin Robertson, pp. 60–76.

Williams A (1974c) The cost | benefit approach. *British Medical Bulletin* **30**: 252–6.

Williams A (1976) *Cost-benefit Analysis in Public Health and Medical Care – comments on a thesis written by Bengt Jönsson.* Lunds Universitet: Nationalekonomiska Institutionen. Meddelande 28 (mimeo, 13p). [Lund University: Department of Economics. Working paper 28 (mimeo 13p).]

Williams A (1977) Health service planning. In: Artis M and Nobay A (eds) *Studies in Modern Economic Analysis: the proceedings of the Association of University Teachers of Economics, Edinburgh 1976.* Oxford: Basil Blackwell & Mott Ltd, pp. 301–35.

Williams A (1981) Welfare Economics and Health Status Measurement. In: J van der Gaag J and Perlman M (eds) *Health, Economics and Health Economics.* Amsterdam: North Holland Publishing, pp. 159–70 and reprinted in: Culyer AJ and Maynard A (eds) (1997) *Being Reasonable about the Economics of Health: selected essays by Alan Williams.* Cheltenham: Edward Elgar Publishing Limited, pp. 107–19.

CHAPTER 4

The public–private challenge in health care

... Alan Maynard

INTRODUCTION

Alan Williams had a phenomenal capacity to teach and mentor, guiding generations of York and non-York colleagues along the paths of enlightenment, a process always based on his maxim: 'Be reasonable! Do it my way!'. I was a grateful beneficiary of his teaching and mentoring over the decades we worked together in York.

He was all too aware of the limitations of finance and delivery in health care, but robust in his defence of a healthcare system based on the principle of need, defined with typical precision as capacity to benefit. At a time when that principle is under renewed challenge in healthcare systems across the world and as diverse as Australia, Canada, and Hong Kong, the purpose of this paper is to elaborate and extend the arguments that Williams deployed about conflicting 'ideals' and 'actuals' in the positions of those holding competing ideologies in the healthcare policy debate. The pertinence of this analysis is increased by the current confused policies of the British government, which, ever anxious to achieve greater efficiency in the use of increased NHS funding, has adopted some innovations whose purposes appear to be inconsistent with the provision of care on the basis of need.

SOCIAL WELFARE FUNCTIONS AND COMPETING IDEOLOGIES

Over 20 years ago, the Thatcher Government was challenging the UK's National Health Service (NHS). The 'social contract' that had governed NHS politics since 1948 had broken down (Klein, 2001). Whereas previously there had been an unwritten concordat by which the medical profession was left to govern the delivery of health care which the government funded, the Thatcher administration increasingly demanded to see evidence of 'value for money'. This implied micromanagement of clinical activity and the doctors' trade union, the British Medical Association, responded by demanding increased funding.

At the same time, and as part of the international and continuous cycle of healthcare reform, the Americans were debating the performance of their own healthcare system. At a conference in Washington DC in 1980, a York trio presented a paper including Williams' description of the attitudes associated with differing ideological viewpoints (Culyer *et al.*, 1981). Williams elaborated this subsequently with descriptions of the actual and idealised characteristics of the competing egalitarian and libertarian healthcare systems (Maynard, 1982; Maynard and Williams, 1984; Williams, 1988).

The three tables from these papers are shown next: attitudes associated with the two viewpoints (Table 4.1), the characteristics of an ideal healthcare system as advocated by adherents to the competing ideologies (Table 4.2), and the nature of the actual competing healthcare systems as critiqued by their opponents (Table 4.3). Adherents of each ideological position tend to criticise the *actual* performance (*see* Table 4.3) of their opponent with the *idealised* characteristics (*see* Table 4.2) of their own system, thereby fuelling rhetorical debate and avoiding addressing the resolution of well-established efficiency and equity deficiencies.

TABLE 4.1 ATTITUDES TYPICALLY ASSOCIATED WITH VIEWPOINTS A AND B

	Viewpoint A (libertarian)	Viewpoint B (egalitarian)
Personal responsibility	Personal responsibility for achievement is very important, but weakened if people are offered unearned rewards. Moreover, they weaken the motive force that assures economic well-being and thereby also undermine moral well-being, because of the intimate connection between moral well-being and the personal effort to achieve.	Personal incentives to achieve are desirable, but economic failure is not equated with moral depravity or social worthlessness.
Social concern	Social Darwinism dictates a seemingly cruel indifference to the fate of those who cannot make the grade.	Private charitable action is not rejected but potentially morally risky (because it may demean the recipient and corrupt the donor) and usually inequitable.

cont.

	Viewpoint A (libertarian)	Viewpoint B (egalitarian)
Social concern (*cont.*)	A less extreme position is that charity, expressed and effected preferably under private auspices, is the proper vehicle, but it needs to be exercised under carefully prescribed conditions: for example, the potential recipient must first mobilise his own resources and, when helped, must be in a less favourable position than the self-supporting (the principle of 'lesser eligibility').	It seems preferable to establish social mechanisms that create and sustain self-sufficiency with precise rules of entitlement that are applied equitably and explicitly sanctioned by society at large.
Freedom	Freedom is sought as a supreme good in itself. Compulsion attenuates both personal responsibility and individualistic and voluntary expressions of social concern. Centralised health planning and a large governmental role in healthcare financing are an unwarranted abridgement of the freedom of both clients and health professionals; private medicine is therefore viewed as a bulwark against totalitarianism.	Freedom is the presence of real opportunities of choice; although economic constraints are less coercive than political constraints, they often represent the effective limits on choice. Freedom is not indivisible but may be sacrificed in one respect in order to obtain greater freedom in another. Government is not an external threat to individuals in society but is the means by which individuals achieve greater scope for action (that is, greater real freedom).
Equality	Equality before the law is the key concept, with clear precedence being given to freedom over equality wherever the two conflict.	Since the only moral justification for using personal achievement as the basis for distributing rewards is that everyone has equal opportunities for such achievement, the main emphasis is on equality of opportunity; where this cannot be assured, the moral worth of achievement is undermined. Equality is the extension to the many of the freedom enjoyed by the few.

Source: This table was published in Williams A (1988) Priority setting in public and private health care: a guide through the ideological jungle. *Journal of Health Economics* **7**: 173–83. Copyright Elsevier, 1988. Used and adapted with permission from Elsevier.

TABLE 4.2 IDEALISED HEALTHCARE SYSTEMS

	Private	Public
Demand	1 Individuals are the best judges of their own welfare.	1 When ill, individuals are frequently imperfect judges of their own welfare.
	2 Priorities determined by own willingness and ability to pay.	2 Priorities determined by social judgements about need.
	3 Erratic and potentially catastrophic nature of demand mediated by private insurance.	3 Erratic and potentially catastrophic nature of demand made irrelevant by provision of free services.
	4 Matters of equity dealt with elsewhere (e.g. in the tax and social security systems).	4 Since the distribution of income and wealth is unlikely to be equitable in relation to the need for health care, the system must be insulated from its influence.
Supply	1 Profit is the proper and effective way to motivate suppliers to respond to demand (need).	1 Professional ethics and dedication to public service are the appropriate motivation, focusing on success in curing or caring.
	2 Priorities determined by people's willingness and ability to pay and by the costs of meeting their wishes at the margin.	2 Priorities determined by where the greatest improvements in caring or curing can be effected at the margin.
	3 Suppliers have strong incentive to adopt least-cost methods of provision.	3 Predetermined limit on available resources generates a strong incentive for suppliers to adopt least-cost methods of provision.
Adjustment mechanism	1 Many competing suppliers ensure that offer prices are kept low and reflect costs.	1 Central review of activities generates efficiency; audit of service provision and management pressures keep the system cost-effective.
	2 Well-informed consumers can seek out the most cost-effective form of treatment.	2 Well-informed clinicians prescribe the most cost-effective form of treatment for each patient.
	3 If, at the price that clears the market, medical practice is profitable, more people will go into medicine and hence supply will be demand responsive.	3 If there is resulting pressure on some facilities or specialties, resources will be directed towards extending them.

cont.

		Private		Public
Adjustment mechanism (*cont.*)	4	If, conversely, medical practice is unprofitable, people will leave it, or stop entering it, until the system returns to equilibrium.	4	Facilities or specialties on which pressure is slack will be slimmed down to release resources for other uses.
Success criteria	1	Consumers judge the system by their ability to achieve what they demand, when, where and how they want it.	1	Electorate judges the system by the extent to which it improves the health status of the population at large in relation to the resources allocated to it.
	2	Producers judge the system by how good a living they make.	2	Producers judge the system by its ability to enable them to provide the treatments they believe to be cost-effective.

Source: This table was published in Williams A (1988) Priority setting in public and private health care: a guide through the ideological jungle. *Journal of Health Economics* **7**: 173–83. Copyright Elsevier, 1988. Used and adapted with permission from Elsevier.

TABLE 4.3 ACTUAL HEALTHCARE SYSTEMS

		Private		Public
Demand	1	Doctors act as agents, mediating demand on behalf of consumers.	1	Doctors act as agents, identifying need on behalf of patients.
	2	Priorities determined by the reimbursement rules of insurance funds.	2	Priorities determined by the doctor's professional situation, his assessment of the patient's condition and the expected trouble-making proclivities of the patient.
	3	Because private insurance coverage is a profit-seeking activity, some risk rating is inevitable; hence, coverage is incomplete and uneven, distorting personal willingness and ability to pay.	3	Absence of direct financial contributions at the point of service and of risk rating enables patients to seek treatment for trivial or inappropriate conditions.
	4	Attempts to change the distribution of income and wealth independently are resisted as destroying incentives (e.g. the ability to buy better or more medical care if you are rich).	4	Attempts to correct inequities in the social and economic system by differential compensatory access to health services may encourage use of health care where it is unlikely to be cost-effective.

cont.

	Private	Public
Supply	1 What is most profitable to suppliers may not reflect consumer interests, and lack of clarity over consumers' interests gives suppliers a range of discretion.	1 Personal professional dedication and public-spirited motivation may degenerate into cynicism if others are seen to be personally benefiting from blatantly self-seeking behaviour.
	2 Priorities determined by the extent to which consumers can be induced to part with their money and by the costs of satisfying the pattern of 'demand'.	2 Priorities determined by what gives the greatest professional satisfaction.
	3 Profit motive strongly incentivises market segmentation and price discrimination and tie-in agreements with other professionals.	3 Since cost-effectiveness is not accepted as a proper medical responsibility, such pressures merely generate tension between the 'professionals' and the 'managers'.
Adjustment mechanism	1 Professional, ethical rules are used to make overt competition difficult.	1 Few elaborate cost data required for billing purposes, so little useful information on costs routinely generated.
	2 Consumers denied information about quality and competence and, since insured, may collude with doctors (against the insurance carriers) in inflating costs.	2 Clinicians know little about costs, have no direct incentive to act on information they have, and sometimes have perverse incentives (i.e. cutting costs may make their life more difficult or less rewarding).
	3 Entry into the profession made difficult and numbers restricted to maintain profitability.	3 Very little known about the relative cost-effectiveness of different treatments and doctors wary of acting on any such information until a general professional consensus emerges.
	4 If demand for services falls, doctors extend range of activities and push out neighbouring disciplines.	4 Phasing out of redundant facilities difficult because it often threatens the livelihood of some concentrated specialised group and has identifiable people dependent on it, whereas beneficiaries are dispersed and only identified as statistics.

cont.

	Private	Public
Success criteria	1 Consumers judge the system by their ability to get someone to do what they need done without making them 'medically indigent' and/or adversely changing their risk rating.	1 Since the easiest aspect of health status to measure is life expectancy, discussion dominated by mortality data and mortality risks to the detriment of treatments concerned with non-life-threatening situations.
	2 Producers judge the system by how good a living they can make out of it.	2 In the absence of accurate data on cost-effectiveness, producers judge the system by the extent to which it enables them to carry out the treatments they find most exciting and satisfying.

Source: This table was published in Williams A (1988) Priority setting in public and private health care: a guide through the ideological jungle. *Journal of Health Economics* **7**: 173–83. Copyright Elsevier, 1988. Used and adapted with permission from Elsevier.

The crux of the distinction between the egalitarian and the libertarian perspectives is the differing maximand in their social welfare functions. The libertarians are concerned with *freedom of choice*, where health care is part of the reward system of society and access to care is determined by willingness and ability to pay. For the egalitarian, the primary focus of concern is *equality of opportunity*. 'Equality is seen as the extension to the many of the freedom enjoyed by only the few' (Culyer *et al.*, 1981). Priorities in an egalitarian system are determined by social judgements about need, where need is defined as the patient's relative ability to benefit in relation to opportunity cost (Williams, 1974).

With adherents of each system subscribing to different social welfare functions, might a 'solution' to their conflict be two co-existing healthcare systems, each serving its own supporters? Unfortunately this is not a viable solution for the egalitarians who view us all as one community with no one opting out. Enhancing the freedom of choice for some, by using market systems and letting individuals exploit their superior purchasing power to shift the distribution of health care in their direction, is inequitable: it gives a higher social priority to more affluent citizens and diminishes social welfare.

Adherents of the egalitarian ideology would welcome a mixed system only if elements of the libertarian system could be shown to enhance the performance of an NHS type. Would some mix of systems do better than either of the systems alone – and what is that mix? For example, can some form of 'competitive market' improve the achievement of NHS goals?

However before addressing such contemporary debates on the supply side issues, the ideological debate on the demand or financing side of the healthcare market will be reviewed.

IDEOLOGY AND THE DEMAND SIDE

The continuous and often repetitive reform debates in all healthcare systems often focus on the demand side of the healthcare market, ignoring the two primary certainties in life: death and the scarcity of resources. Depending on the state of the world economy, reformers from the left and right assert that systems are either 'too expensive' or 'underfunded'. For example, expenditure in the US health systems and in private insurance systems generally inflates at two to three times that of the consumer price index (Colombo and Tapay, 2004) and the left proffer National Health Insurance as the solution (Emanuel and Fuchs, 2005). In 'socialised' healthcare systems, the problem is asserted to be 'underfunding' where libertarians typically advocate user charges as a 'solution' and the left advocates spending more, as in Blair's UK reforms.

The drivers of expenditure in healthcare systems are technological advance, the ageing of the population and the effects of these factors and increasing gross domestic product (GDP) on public expectations. Market and socialised healthcare systems are quite poor at managing these pressures. Technology appraisal is slowly inserting economic evaluation into public decision making, but notions of opportunity cost and budget constraints remain poorly defined, thereby allowing innovations of marginal cost-effectiveness to be imposed on healthcare managers. The effects of ageing may be moderated by the predicted compression of morbidity (Fries *et al.*, 1989), but the evidence of such effects is the subject of lively debate (Manton *et al.*, 1997; Jacobzone *et al.*, 2000). Even if compression of morbidity is modest or absent, the cost 'burden' of this triumph of extending people's lives may be modest. Those concerned with the effects of ageing and profit-driven technology marketeers propound, in their various ways, the nirvana of immortality when the evidence base for the majority of healthcare interventions is absent (BMJ Publishing Group, 2005) and many practices may be little more than expensive placebos!

Debates such as these about the drivers of expenditure do not drive public policy. Instead, special cases and well-marketed advocacy lead to a focus on how increased funding will be financed, raising ideological and distributional issues (*see* Boxes 4.1–4.3).

The libertarian perspective, currently epitomised by Bush in the USA, Howard in Australia and reform proposals in Hong Kong, prefer private insurance, user charges and medical savings accounts (MSAs). MSAs are family-based insurance systems that first emerged in Singapore and a number of large Chinese cities. Wage earners are obliged to contribute and usually subsidised to save in order to fund the healthcare costs of extended family members, i.e. the risk pool is small. These devices obviously advantage the affluent whose saving capacity is greater, and the tax subsidies augment inequalities. In Singapore MSAs fund only about 10% of total expenditure and there, and in mainland China, they have been shown to increase inequalities and brought few observable efficiency gains, instead often increasing provider

BOX 4.1 FINANCING IN AUSTRALIA

In Australia, the Howard Government has increased private insurance cover in by tax subsidies, by lifetime savings accounts, which 'buy in' the young at low levels of premium, and increased taxation of those who do not hold private healthcare insurance. His antipathy to Australian Medicare, a national system of healthcare provision, reduces the tax revenues by $A2.5 billion, which benefits the more affluent (Hall and Maynard, 2005). These policies are articulated in terms of 'freedom' and Howard's lifelong antipathy to 'socialised' health care. It has helped him to be re-elected three times and will be difficult to reverse if an egalitarian government ever re-emerges.

BOX 4.2 FINANCING IN HONG KONG

In Hong Kong, the healthcare spend is modest, consuming less than 6% of GDP. Hospital care is provided in a mini-NHS, which is tax financed. Primary care is provided largely by the private sector, physicians make a fine living from work in this office-based and poorly regulated system, and access is based on ability to pay. The 'communist' government's response to expenditure problems has been to advocate the increased use of private insurance and medical savings accounts (MSAs) (Health, Welfare and Food Bureau, 2004), primarily as tax levels are believed to be 'too high' (income tax is 14%). Income inequality in Hong Kong is considerable, and its perpetuation by the 'communist' libertarian government is seen as essential to maintain high levels of economic growth.

profits and the use of often unproven high technology (Yip and Hsiao, 1997; Yi *et al.*, 2005).

Perhaps unsurprisingly, Bush has implemented a version of MSAs in the USA.

Another familiar weapon in the libertarian armoury is the advocacy of user charges. This was the preferred policy in the USA in the 1980s and was supplanted by evidence-free optimism about 'managed care' in the 1990s. While managed care may have moderated healthcare expenditure inflation in the mid-1990s with no apparent quality consequences, there was a 'bounce back' as providers used market power to countervail funders' purchasing power, reviving high inflation rates. The policy response to this is the re-adoption of the failed policies of the 1980s, i.e. deductibles, co-insurance and manipulation of benefit package coverage.

Stoddart and his colleagues have reviewed the literature on user charges several times. They reiterate each time their conclusions:

> In the present structure of health care delivery, most proposals for 'patient participation in health care financing' reduce to misguided or cynical efforts to tax the ill and/or drive up the total cost of health care while shifting some of the burden out of government budgets.
>
> (Stoddart *et al.*, 1993, pp. 25, 37)

Of course these authors are coming from an egalitarian perspective. User charges for libertarians empower consumers to express their freedom of choice, and they have less concern about the equity consequences of 'taxing' the ill, who are also often poor and elderly. As Stoddart notes, such instruments may also increase expenditure, with the asymmetry of market information facilitating supplier-induced demand.

The cycle of advocacy of changes in healthcare funding in socialised systems represents a continuing attempt by libertarians to undermine the egalitarian structures of healthcare finance. Often this advocacy of funding reform is accompanied by arguments that demand cannot be funded alone from tax/social insurance finance, even though such 'single-pipe' funding is a necessary, if not sufficient condition for healthcare expenditure control, and that the instruments advocated by libertarians are unlikely to produce efficiency gains (*see* Tables 4.2 and 4.3). Nevertheless much sound and fury is spent on what is, in effect, an irrelevant debate for egalitarians.

However the mutual posturing of both sides of such debates appears to serve a purpose which is utility generating for each participant, i.e. with policy focused on the largely irrelevant demand/funding side, everyone can ignore supply-side inefficiencies which for decades have been well evidenced and maintained by a conspiracy of silence.

IDEOLOGY AND THE SUPPLY SIDE

Whatever the nature of the organisation of a healthcare system, all appear to exhibit a common problem: a reluctance to deal with well-evidenced supply-side failures in terms of healthcare process and outcome. Let us briefly review these problems: the application of the evidence base, the ubiquitous nature of clinical practice variation, and the absence of outcome measurement and management.

The application of the evidence base

Firstly it is evident that despite the work of the Cochrane Collaboration, a considerable portion of medicine has no evidence base. The James Lind Alliance aims to establish partnerships between patients and clinicians to identify and prioritise current uncertainties about medical practice and to ensure that they inform future research agendas. One product of the Lind alliance is a Database of Uncertainties about the Effectiveness of Treatments (DUETs, accessible at www.duets.nhs.uk). The extent of the uncertainty about clinical effectiveness is considerable (*see* Figure 4.1).

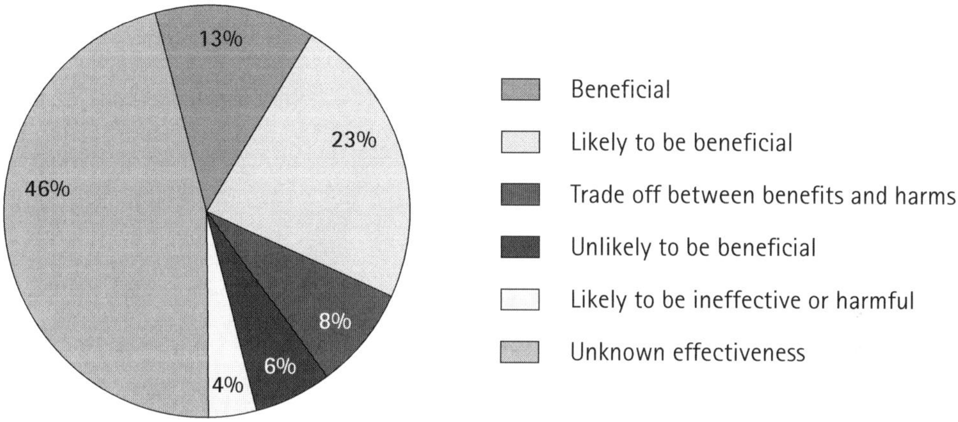

FIGURE 4.1 Uncertainty about clinical effectiveness. *Source*: Figure taken from the BMJ Clinical Evidence website 'About us' section, www.clinicalevidence.com [accessed 5 September 2007]. Used with permission from the BMJ Publishing Group Ltd.

Such information is pertinent when investing in medical care. However, the important issue is that evidence-based treatments are not delivered to patients, thereby increasing morbidity and mortality. This is particularly the case for the chronically ill, where there are established ways of identifying patients in need, and relatively cheap and cost-effective treatments, although side-effects may affect compliance. Universally we can see evidence of this. For example, in the USA where 16% of a large GDP is spent on health care, Americans allegedly get only 55% of appropriate care (Kerr *et al.*, 2004). Similar problems can be seen in most developed countries, middle-income countries such as China and Egypt, and low-income countries such as Kyrgyzstan.

In Britain, one policy response to this problem is the QOF in the 2004 contract for primary care (*see* Box 4.3). Despite the defects of the QOF, it is a notable attempt to remedy a long-term problem of failure to implement interventions of proven efficacy and it can be improved over time. Parallel attempts in the USA have generally been feeble, with report systems being used on a voluntary basis by insurers and managed care companies, with some participants insisting that their responses are confidential. 'Competitive' markets and commercial incentives do not improve compliance in the absence of regulation!

BOX 4.3 PRIMARY CARE INNOVATIONS IN BRITAIN

The Quality and Outcomes Framework (QOF), introduced to NHS general practice in 2004, is based on 'points' collected by practices for meeting various clinical and organisational targets. This largely rewards primary care practices for doing what they *should* have been doing anyway and is deemed a 'success' by government, as achievement levels of 91% have exceeded planned targets of 75%. This success is ambiguous as there are no 'before' data to compare with the 'after' achievement levels. Further, the evidence base for the 10 clinical activities targeted by generous fee-for-service incentives has been criticised (Fleetcroft and Cookson, 2006), and the weighting between the categories appears to reflect not their relative clinical importance in terms of improving population health but the estimated workload for GP practices.

Variations in clinical practice

With so little in medicine certain and supported by the evidence base, it is unsurprising that different clinicians treat similar patients in very different ways! Clinical practice variation has been the subject of considerable analysis for decades, and remarkably this evidence has had very little impact on practice and policy: the inefficiencies are well recognised by libertarians and egalitarians, both of whom have failed to mitigate them with effective supply-side reforms.

For example, in the US, Jack Wennberg and his colleagues at the Dartmouth Medical School have carried out the most sustained and insightful of this work. For over two decades this group has analysed Medicare data, initially comparing similar areas (e.g. New Haven and Boston) and more recently charting the geographical variations across the country (Wennberg *et al.*, 1987, 1989). For instance US Medicare spending per capita in 2000 was $10 550 per enrolee in Manhattan and $4823 in Portland, Oregon. The differences were ascribed to volume effects rather than illness differences, socio-economic status or the price of services. Fisher summarised this work as follows:

> Residents in high spending regions received 60% more but did not have lower mortality rates, better functional status or higher satisfaction.
>
> (Fisher, 2003)

He went on to suggest that potential savings of 30% of the Medicare budget were possible if high spenders reduced expenditure and provided the safe practices of conservative treatment areas.

Recently in England as the government became frustrated by the reluctance of the NHS to follow the Prime Minister's dictum and 'act smarter', academic research and government agencies, in particular the Modernisation Agency and its successor the NHS Institute for Innovation have again emphasised the scope for 'efficiency savings'. For instance the work of Bloor, who used routine NHS Hospital Episode Statistics to identify significant differences in consultant activity measured in terms of volume (finished consultant episodes or FCEs) and in terms of 'value' (i.e. volume multiplied by Healthcare Resource Group (HRG) price), was an input into debates within the Department of Health about the adoption of fee-for-service payments to consultants as a means of shifting the modest mean of this distribution and reducing dispersion. However, these data had little impact on an NHS that continues to use its own routine data to inform management by clinicians and non-clinicians (Bloor and Maynard, 2002, 2006).

One current focus of UK NHS reform is improving knowledge and management of variations in the adoption of proven technologies and reducing variations in clinical practice. This is remarkably reminiscent of the efforts of the Wilson Labour Government 30 years ago. The then Department of Health and Social Security (DHSS) sought to get the NHS to focus on the evidence base for day case surgery and the reduction of variations in clinical practice (DHSS, 1976). The failure of 30 years of NHS 'redisorganisations' of structures to alter clinical processes is noticeable!

The absence of outcome measurement and management

Williams dedicated his life to persuading reformers, clinical and political, to the cause of patient reported outcomes measures (PROM). Whilst he had some success in getting such quantification into health technology assessment, in particular the use of QALYs in the National Institute for Health and Clinical Excellence (NICE), one of his final papers (Kind and Williams, 2004) again emphasised the absence of routine PROM measurement and management in the NHS. There are now signs that policy makers may invest in PROM and the measurement of, for instance, physical and mental functioning before and after elective procedures in the NHS. This could revolutionise the management of medical practice by making clinical activity more transparent as well as facilitating systematic appraisal of the success of the NHS in improving health.

IDEOLOGY AND ADJUSTMENT MECHANISMS: HEALTHCARE REFORM

The libertarian and egalitarian protagonists engaged in ideological battles for healthcare reform focus on the 'ideal' characteristics of the adjustment mechanism (*see* Table 4.2), even though the 'actual' nature of their systems are well defined (*see* Table 4.3). The failure of both models to produce efficient outcomes is a product of the incentives facing both consumers and providers.

In egalitarian systems, and ignoring the largely irrelevant arguments for funding changes proffered by libertarians, the usual focus of reform is the use of 'competition' in either the management of funds and/or the delivery of services. Thus, in countries such as the Netherlands and Switzerland, 'choice' of insuring sickness fund is seen as an essential part of using competition to improve resource allocation. Whether these measures improve choice and the efficiency of service delivery for patients is unclear (Herzlinger and Parsa-Parsi, 2004; Reinhardt, 2004; Schut and Van de Ven, 2005).

One lesson to be learnt from this literature is the need for careful regulation of competition and the integration of each component part of the reform package so that they are complementary rather than conflicting. This is nicely epitomised by the Dutch approach to competition, and in Enthoven's advocacy of regulated competition. In the latter's Jackson Hole reform proposals for the USA (Ellwood *et al.*, 1992), there was to be regulation of premium setting for competing insurers, definition of a basic package, which was to be guaranteed to the less affluent through tax subsidies, and regulation to ensure both health technology appraisal and the national measurement of outcomes. These structures aimed to ensure risk spreading in the insurance system and to control the supplier-induced demand excesses of doctors. Regulation in the Dutch system includes risk-related premiums so that competing insurers are not disadvantaged by having disproportionate numbers of poor risks, and with detailed regulation of the supply side including anti-trust regulation to break up provider cartels.

The careful articulation of a regulatory framework in these schemes contrasts with the Blair Government's conversion to 'constructive discomfort' (Stevens, 2004) and contestability in market structures in the English NHS. Here a series of radical innovations has preceded the construction of a regulatory framework. This 'cart before the horse' approach has created financial instability and associated media pressure about the 'failure' of the Blair reforms. Underlying this controversy is a fundamental issue related again to the choice of ideology, i.e. is the goal of policy to create a demand-led NHS or one based as in the past, on need?

This clash of objectives is epitomised by the tariffs policy (known in Britain as 'payment by results' (PbR), but similar to diagnostic-related groups (DRGs) in other systems). The issue here is the role of PbR in a cash-limited, public insurance/NHS system. In 2006–2007 tariffs are determining 80% of hospital income. For elective procedures there is a set of tariffs with no cap. For emergency procedures the full tariff is paid only for volume up to 2004–2005 levels plus 3%, after which the tariff is reduced by 50%. However again there is no cap and a 50% tariff can be attractive for hospitals operating at marginal cost. Those hospitals with capacity and costs below the PbR average have a clear incentive to trade up, while those with higher costs have to meet access targets and are also incentivised to increase throughput and maximise income. Unsurprisingly, meeting local demand in this way contributes to expenditure exceeding budgets.

However, local budgets are determined by a weighted capitation formula that reflects local need through crude proxies such as mortality and pertinent, selected measures of deprivation. Initially the product of the Resource Allocation Working Party (RAWP) in 1977, geographical inequalities in financial capacity to meet need have been narrowed. PbR has contributed a major disruption to this, with deficits for 2005–2006 exceeding £1.2 billion. To cap PbR would however disrupt another government policy, foundation hospitals. These free-standing providers trade on the basis of legally enforceable contracts and with PbR tariffs. Current policy to resolve these issues emphasises financial balance and ignores the incentives created by fragmented reforms.

Another controversial policy in Britain is the use of the private sector as a provider and, in the near future, as a commissioner of health care. In order to create uncertainty and augment capacity to hit elective waiting time targets (Stevens, 2004), the government has contracted private providers who are typically paid at PbR rates plus a premium of 15% to encourage market entry. While such providers appear to be exploiting both economies of scale (e.g. purchasing limited ranges of prostheses) and tighter clinical pathways, it is inevitable that they cream-skim, e.g. taking routine hip and knee cases, leaving the NHS with complex patients and revisions. In primary care, only one general practice in Derbyshire has been 'privatised' to date, with United Health of the USA contracted to provide local NHS care.

Those with an egalitarian perspective want the public sector to be stronger and the private sector weaker because they are concerned that social solidarity will be undermined, allowing the affluent and the articulate to opt out. This threat can be minimised if the regulatory framework is robust and efficient, which is not the case in the current NHS, as private entities are contracted to carry out some NHS activities. However, there is a risk that such work will produce profits from NHS funding that will be used to advantage private patients, and that once private entities have a share of NHS business, they may exploit this through the legislative processes.

As Williams argued, there is scope to learn managerial techniques from other systems. However (he argued), 'I observe that many of the supposed "improvements" in "efficiency" contain implications about priority setting in health care which seem to me to have a quite strong (though implicit) ideological component and which I feel bound to reject because of their distributional implications' (Williams, 1988).

IDEOLOGY AND CRITERIA FOR SUCCESS

As Williams would have argued, the crucial ingredient absent so far in the discussion of demand and supply-side failures is patient outcomes, i.e. do clinical interventions improve patients' mental and physical functioning? As he remarked, it is strange how the medical profession usurped the role of economists in being 'dismal scientists' with their focus on failure indicators such as mortality, complications and readmissions, while our 'noble profession', at least the *health* economists, wished to focus on success and the improvement of the patient's health status! His innovative work on outcomes with colleagues such as Paul Kind tackled what is an old problem.

The Babylonians were clearly interested in what the Americans now call P4P, or payment for performance; this 'health indicator' can now be found in the Louvre:

> If a surgeon has made a deep incision in the body of a man with a lancet of bronze and saves the man's life, or has opened an abscess in the eye of a man and has saved his eye, he shall take 10 shekels of silver. If the surgeon has made a deep incision in the body of a man with a lancet of bronze and so destroys the man's eye, they shall cut off his forehand.
>
> (Rosser, 1983, p. 50)

Subsequent generations of physicians have advocated the systematic recording of activity and success including Thomas Percival (1740–1804), a Warrington practitioner who wrote a pamphlet on the internal regulation of hospitals in 1771, the editor of the *Lancet* in 1841, who repeated the advocacy of Francis Clifton, physician to George I in the previous century, by calling for systematic data collection and management, and EA Codman, an early 20th century product of Harvard, who lost his staff privileges in 1914 when Massachusetts General Hospital refused to institute his plan for evaluating the competence of surgeons. Codman was an advocate of an 'end result system of hospital standardisation'.

Percival in 1803 argued:

> By the adoption of the register, physicians and surgeons would obtain clearer insight into the comparative success of their hospital and private practice; and would be incited to diligent investigation of the cause of such difference.*

Codman in 1914 argued:

> Every hospital should follow every patient it treats long enough to determine whether the treatment has been successful, and then to inquire 'if not, why not?', with a view to preventing similar failures in the future.†

And finally, Kind and Williams in 2004:

> It is remarkable that we know so little about the health improvements brought about by the enormous array of activities provided by the NHS . . . the routine monitoring of outcomes has yet to be tackled in a systematic way.
>
> (Kind and Williams, 2004, p. 1)

* www.thornber.net/cheshire/ideasmen/percival.html

† www.whonamedit.com/doctor.cfm/2558.html

While Florence Nightingale's advocacy of 'dead, relieved and unrelieved' as outcome measures (Nightingale, 1863) had some temporary impact in the 19th century and, prior to the establishment of the NHS in 1948, especially in psychiatric hospitals where such monitoring was obligatory, the last three decades have seen the proliferation of generic and specific quality-of-life measures, their translation into dozens of languages and their application in thousands of clinical trials, but an absence of their routine use in clinical practice.

Thus a necessary criterion for measuring and managing the success of the competing ideologies, namely applying existing generic and specific patient-reported outcome measures (PROM) in routine primary and secondary care, is absent. How that could be incentivised is a nice issue, e.g. obliging commissioners to contract on the basis of PROM performance and incorporating routine PROM assessments in primary care via the QOF. Without such incentives, the measurement of success will focus on limited measures of failure (e.g. cardiothoracic surgical mortality rates, where technology (e.g. stents and statins) may make the procedure redundant!), and the policy debate will return to futile arguments about funding and access targets, which alone are of limited relevance.

CONCLUSIONS

Williams' exposition of libertarian and egalitarian viewpoints clarifies the differing maxims in their social welfare functions: libertarians are concerned primarily with freedom of choice, and egalitarians with equality of opportunity (perhaps in health care, with equality of access). Recent research has shown that what patients in England want is not so much choice, but quality (Burge *et al.*, 2006). Choice in the English NHS, (surely a means to an end and not an end in itself?), is one of a range of government reforms that need careful scrutiny by adherents to the competing ideologies. Like PbR, private sector competition and foundation trusts in Britain, choice may have distributive consequences that thwart egalitarian goals. Choice appears largely irrelevant for emergency and chronically ill patients, who want a guarantee of local quality in healthcare delivery. The other reforms may distort local priorities and reduce the equity of the NHS. For those of an egalitarian perspective they are disruptive, although for the libertarians they represent the sighting of a distant oasis where freedom of choice may reign and resources are allocated on the basis of willingness and ability to pay!

The purpose of each of these reforms is to improve efficiency, although evidence of their success in achieving this goal is poor. Their success in upholding egalitarian principles will depend not just on their marginality, so they act as temporary catalysts for needed improvements in resource allocation, but also on their regulation within a coherent framework that measures and manages success. Both these conditions appear to be absent at present in England.

The internal reform of egalitarian systems such as the NHS requires both improved measurement of outcomes, a subject close to Williams' heart, and incentives that address clinical and cost-effectiveness uncertainty, the variations in clinical practice that result from this uncertainty, and the clinical 'discretion' which protects variation and the reluctance of doctors to measure and manage patient-reported outcomes.

As Williams outlined, adherents of each ideological position tend to criticise the actual performance of their opponent with the idealised characteristics of their own system. The objectives of healthcare systems and reforms are typically cost containment, equity and efficiency, but these objectives often conflict, and the priority assigned to each differs with economic and political cycles. In Britain, the strengths of tax-based egalitarian systems (cost containment and equality of access) remain, but attempts to improve efficiency (using techniques derived from more libertarian systems) have potential to undermine both objectives. The appropriate balance in healthcare systems of public and private, of choice and equality, and of equity and efficiency, is still determined largely by ideological debates, but should increasingly be informed by hard evidence, particularly on patient-reported health outcomes.

REFERENCES

Bloor K and Maynard A (2002) Consultants: managing them means measuring them. *Health Service Journal* **112**: 10–11.

Bloor K and Maynard A (2006) Consultant clinical activity is key to improving productivity. *Health Service Journal* **116**: 18–19.

BMJ Publishing Group (2005) *British Medical Journal: clinical evidence concise*. London: BMJ Publishing. www.clinicalevidence.com (accessed 7 March 2007).

Burge P, Devlin N, Appleby J *et al.* (2006) *Understanding Patients' Choices at the Point of Referral.* RAND Europe Working Paper. London: King's Fund. www.kingsfund.org.uk/document.rm?id=6438 (accessed 7 March 2007).

Colombo F and Tapay N. (2004) *Private Health Insurance in OECD. Benefits and costs of individuals and health systems*. OECD Health Working Papers: 15. Paris: OECD Directorate for Employment, Labour and Social Affairs.

Culyer AJ, Maynard A and Williams A (1981) Alternative systems of health care provision: an essay on motes and beams. In: Olson M (ed.) *A New Approach to the Economics of Health Care*. Washington DC: American Enterprise Institute, pp. 131–50.

Department of Health and Social Security (1976) *Priorities for Health and Personal Social Services in England: a consultation document.* London: HMSO.

Ellwood PM, Enthoven A and Etheridge L (1992) The Jackson Hole initiatives for a twenty-first century American health care system. *Health Economics* **1**: 149–68.

Emanuel EJ and Fuchs V (2005) Health care vouchers: a proposal for universal coverage. *New England Journal of Medicine* **352**: 1255–60.

Fisher ES (2003) Medical care: is more always better? *New England Journal of Medicine* **349**: 1665–7.

Fleetcroft R and Cookson R (2006) Do incentive payments in the new NHS contract for primary care reflect likely population health gains? *Journal of Health Services Research and Policy*, **11**: 27–31.

Fries JF, Green LW and Levine S (1989) Health promotion and the compression of morbidity. *Lancet* **1**: 481–3.

Hall J and Maynard A (2005) Health care lessons from Australia: what can Michael Howard learn from John Howard? *British Medical Journal* **330**: 357–9.

Health, Welfare and Food Bureau (2004) *Studies on Health Care Financing and Feasibility of a Medical Savings Scheme in Hong Kong*. Discussion Paper CB(2)2692/03-04(03). www.hwfb.gov.hk/hmdac/english/dis_papers/dis_papers_hcfppd.html (accessed 7 March 2007).

Herzlinger RE and Parsa-Parsi R (2004) Consumer-driven health care: lessons from Switzerland. *Journal of the American Medical Association* **292**: 1213–20.

Jacobzone S, Cambois E and Robine JM. (2000) Is the health of older persons in OECD countries improving enough to compensate for population ageing? *OECD Economic Studies* **30**: 149–90.

Kind P and Williams A. (2004) *Measuring Success in Healthcare – the time has come to do it properly. University of York, Health Policy Matters* March, issue 9. www.york.ac.uk/healthsciences/pubs/HPM9final.pdf (accessed 7 March 2007).

Kerr EA, McGlynn EA, Adams J Keesey J and SM Asch (2004) Profiling the quality of care in twelve communities: results from the CQI study. *Health Affairs* **23**: 247–56.

Klein R (2001) *The new politics of the NHS* (4e). Harlow: Prentice Hall.

Manton KG, Corder L and Stallard E (1997) Chronic disability trends in elderly US populations, 1982–1994. *Proceedings of the National Academy of Sciences of the USA* **94**: 2593–8.

Maynard A (1982) The regulation of public and private health care markets. In: McLachlan G and Maynard A (eds) *The Public Private Mix for Health*. London: Nuffield Provincial Hospitals Trust, pp. 471–511.

Maynard A and Williams A (1984) Privatisation and the NHS. In: Le Grand J and Robinson R (eds), *Privatisation and the Welfare State*. London: Allen and Unwin, pp. 95–110.

Nightingale F (1863) *Notes on Hospitals*. London: Longman, Green, Longman, Roberts and Green.

Reinhardt UE (2004) The Swiss health care system: regulated competition without managed care. *Journal of the American Medical Association* **292**: 1227–31.

Rosser R (1983) A history of the development of health indicators. In: Teeling Smith G (ed.) *Measuring the Social Benefits of Medicare*. London: Office of Health Economics, pp. 50–62.

Schut FT and Van de Ven WP (2005) Rationing and competition in the Dutch health care system. *Health Economics* **14**(Suppl. 1): 59–75.

Stevens S (2004) Reform Strategies for the English NHS. *Health Affairs* **23(3)**: 37–44.

Stoddart GL, Barer M and Evans R (1993) *User Charges, Snares and Delusions. Another look at the literature*. Vancouver: Centre for Health Services and Policy Research, University of British Columbia.

Wennberg JE, Freeman JL and Culp WJ (1987) Are hospital services rationed in New Haven or over-utilised in Boston? *Lancet* **1**: 1185–9.

Wennberg JE, Freeman JL, Shelton RM and Bubolz TA (1989) Hospital use and mortality among Medicare beneficiaries in Boston and New Haven. *New England Journal of Medicine* **321**: 1168–73.

Williams A (1974) 'Need' as a demand concept (with special reference to health). In: Culyer A (ed). *Economic Policies and Social Goods*. London: Martin Robertson, pp. 60–76.

Williams A (1988) Priority setting in public and private health care: a guide through the ideological jungle. *Journal of Health Economics* 7: 173–83.

Yi Y, Maynard A, Liu G, Xiong X and Lin F (2005) Equity in health care financing: evaluation of the current urban employee health insurance reform in China. *Journal of the Asia Pacific Economy* **10**: 506–27.

Yip WC and Hsiao WC (1997) Medical savings accounts: lessons from China. *Health Affairs* **16**: 244–51.

CHAPTER 5

Discussion of Alan Maynard's paper: 'The public–private challenge in health care'

... Dominique Polton

Discussing priority setting in public and private health care, Alan Williams outlined the conceptions of healthcare systems associated with two competing ideologies: the libertarian ideology, which emphasises freedom and personal responsibility, and views health and access to health care as part of the reward system; and the egalitarian ideology, based on equal opportunity of access to health care, independently of income (Williams, 1988). They have polarised views on demand (demand-driven system versus priorities determined by social judgment about need), supply (profit versus professional ethic and financial constraint as incentives), adjustment mechanisms (market versus central planning and management pressures) and criteria of success (consumers versus citizens).

Interestingly, Alan Williams highlighted the gap between the idealised functioning of these two healthcare systems, as advocated by their adherents, and the way they work in practice. In private systems, market failures in the healthcare sector distort competition; in public systems, the supposed benevolent regulator tends to satisfy professional corporations and the immediate expectations of the population at the expense of cost-effective choices.

HEALTHCARE REFORMS INSPIRED BY A LIBERTARIAN IDEOLOGY

Alan Maynard uses this framework to analyse the ongoing reforms in various healthcare systems. He argues that these reforms are more inspired by a libertarian ideology than by evidence, notably reforms based on the regulation of demand through financial responsibility of individuals – as in the US, Australia or Hong Kong. Even in egalitarian health care systems where this notion of increased financial responsibility is set aside, competition and choice tend to be viewed as solutions in themselves, leading to controversial policies as in the English NHS, such as increasing use of the private sector and reform of hospital tariffs policy.

There seems indeed to be a general libertarian trend in healthcare systems. Since the beginning of the 1990s, the idea of introducing or reinforcing market forces in the healthcare sector has spread in countries with very different initial designs. In a country like the US, which was already largely reliant upon a private insurance market, competition increased during the managed care era. Competition for enrolees between sickness funds has now been the rule in the Netherlands and Germany for more than a decade. The Netherlands has gone one step further with the 2006 reform, extending competition between private insurance funds for the whole population. Other trends include questioning the legitimacy of government rationing of health care and pressure for private funding to complement public coverage (e.g. the Supreme Court decision about private health insurance in Québec).

Most of these planned or implemented reforms tend to be designed on ideological grounds. The belief is spreading that elements of economic liberalism will solve the problems faced by healthcare systems, although this belief is not supported by evidence. For example, one of the expected outcomes of competition between insurers is enhanced competition between providers: in that respect, the evolution of the US system should lead to caution. The failure of the managed care as a structural solution to regulate the healthcare system was in part inherent to its dynamic, and shows the drawbacks of this type of competition. The system that has emerged from this failure is ever more individualistic, with the development of consumer-driven health plans and health-saving accounts (Polton, 2004).

The libertarian trend is also evident in the old European egalitarian systems. Whether it actually undermines the equity principles of these systems is debatable. A close analysis of four countries where elements of managed competition have been introduced (Belgium, Germany, the Netherlands and Switzerland) concluded that the impact was mixed, and found evidence of increased solidarity due to health insurance reform (which was sometimes an explicit aim) (Maarse and Paulus, 2003). One of the reasons is that despite their egalitarian inspiration, most European systems have historically allowed unequal treatment of populations through various mechanisms: professional fragmentation, incomplete coverage, exemption of the richest part of the population from public insurance, or opportunity to opt out or to get supplementary coverage etc. Thus so far there has been scope for improvements of solidarity, or explicit policies for reducing health inequalities, while introducing market-like elements such as prospective reimbursement, increase of private payments or competition between insurers or providers. However, it is necessary to monitor these developments carefully and to ensure that the equity objectives are preserved, in practice as well as in principle.

If these reforms are based more on ideology than on evidence, then what would be an evidence-based policy to cope with the difficulties of all health systems – i.e. tensions between pressures to increase expenditures and public finance constraints, conflicting objectives of efficiency, equity, user satisfaction and cost control?

TACKLING THE SUPPLY-SIDE INEFFICIENCIES AS THE OBVIOUS SOLUTION

According to Alan Maynard, the obvious and straightforward solution is to tackle supply-side inefficiencies, which have been known for decades. On the contrary, the libertarian approach focuses on irrelevant issues of demand and funding. Indeed, the libertarians endorse the argument that healthcare expenditures will inevitably grow to justify regressive policies of increasing individual financial responsibility, although the real impact of these drivers of expenditures and their ineluctability are questionable.

I will argue that the funding and demand aspects cannot be so easily dismissed and need a real debate, taking into account that the real world is one of mixed systems. On the other hand, gaining efficiency on the supply side is invariably a very complicated process with modest achievements and very imperfect tools.

The funding of healthcare systems: a false debate?

The starting point of Alan Maynard's demonstration is that the inevitability of expenditure increase is a false premise – and explains the focus on the question of how to finance the necessary funding (a frequent answer being to raise user charges, given public budget constraints). He argues that the alleged drivers of expenditures have less impact than is often argued (e.g. the ageing of the population), or that they result in an inefficient use of resources (e.g. technological change).

The ageing of the population

In contrast to the popular and journalistic view, health economists have repeatedly argued that the ageing of the population has in itself a limited impact on healthcare expenditures, because this process of change in the demographic structure is slow, as the nice metaphor used by Robert Evans (glacier or avalanche) suggests (Barer and Evans, 1995). The growing share of expenditures going to the elderly population is mainly the result of a drift in the health expenditure age profile, which is due not to higher morbidity, but to changes in practices and technological innovation (Dormont *et al.*, 2006).

However the impact of ageing, even limited, will increase over the next decades (in variable proportions depending on the country), and will require extra funding, while other needs of the elderly population (pensions, long-term care) will put a growing pressure on the working population.

In addition, as Alan acknowledges, the debate on the evolution of health status associated with longevity (compression or expansion of morbidity) is ongoing. There is mixed evidence and uncertainty for the future: the hypothesis of an increased burden of chronic diseases, such as diabetes, in a growing elderly population cannot be excluded.

Technological advance

Alan Maynard argues that if new technologies put a pressure on healthcare expenditures, many are of no value in terms of health outcome: 'the evidence base for a majority of healthcare interventions is absent and many practices may be little more than expensive placebos'. Following this line of reasoning, resisting the pressure of the lobbies on the supply side to introduce pseudo-technological advance and dispensing with ineffective care which brings no benefits to the population should be sufficient, without having to raise the issue of extra funding in health care.

However this argument is debatable, and Alan Williams himself expressed an opposite view:

> Both systems [i.e. public and private] have then to face the problem that the recent rapid growth of effective health care has led us to the point where no country (not even the richest) can afford to carry out all the potentially beneficial procedures that are now available, on all the people who might possibly benefit from them. So priority setting can no longer simply be a matter of eliminating ineffective activities . . . Priority setting now has to deal with the much more contentious high level efficiency problem of choosing where to be on the production possibility frontier, that is which mix of efficient activities to select from those that are open to us.
>
> (Williams, 1988)

The demand for health and health care

Another controversial point concerns the demand for health care. The widely held view of 'infinite demand' obviously serves the interests of those who benefit from increased spending, as Alan Maynard points out. The health industry is indeed eager to endorse the view that health care is a luxury good, prone to grow faster than income, and some economists support this position: in France, a couple of years ago, a think tank of economists published a report defending the idea that policies rationing health care were nonsense and that the only legitimate limit was on public financing of these expenditures (Le Cercle des Économistes, 2004).

On the other hand, other economists have shown that there is no such thing as a demand for health care, in the sense of a classical demand function in economic theory (Rice, 1998). The widespread idea that health care is a luxury good has also been challenged: it is generally based on the observation that the share of health expenditures in GDP is positively linked with GDP. But further research has shown that this elasticity may not be greater than one when other variables are taken into account (Gerdtham and Jönsson, 2000).

Besides, a relationship at the societal level reflects collective choices, which is different from individual choices.

Again, Alan Williams enlightens this issue in showing that although economists are very reluctant to use the concept of 'need', they cannot totally avoid it in health care, where the demand cannot play the role it plays in other sectors (Williams, 1974).

However, the fact that the mere confrontation of supply and demand is not the proper mechanism to determine the level of health insurance and health care consumed, as it is in other markets, does not mean that there is no demand for health care in the general sense, and no preference for health care over other desirable goods. People may prefer to use extra income to improve access to care, perhaps through public coverage. The question is of course which mechanism should be used to elicit preferences, which cannot derive from individual decisions of sovereign consumers, and should reflect democratic choices. But there is no reason to exclude *a priori* an increase of funding for health care from these choices.

For all these reasons, the issues of demand and extra funding are not irrelevant. The question is: how should a potential increase of healthcare expenditures be financed?

If more funding is necessary or desirable, how should it be organised?

For pedagogic purposes, we often use typified situations and simplify reality in order to conceptualise it. In this sense, the opposition between the libertarian and egalitarian views is helpful. But in practice, a totally libertarian system does not exist: even countries such as the US, who rely strongly on market forces, had to ensure access to health care for high-risk and low-income people who would not have been covered by private insurance. Nor does a totally egalitarian system exist: none of our European systems is purely public or egalitarian, as all allow some private funding and/or private insurance.

In some countries, public and private insurance cover separate populations, e.g. in the Netherlands before the 2006 reform, with 30% of the population (i.e. those with higher income) being covered by private insurance; to a lesser extent, the same is true in Germany. In other countries, private insurance buys goods and services that are excluded from public coverage (such as drugs or dental care). Elsewhere, private insurance allows access to providers that are not funded through public insurance, as in the UK (private hospitals). In some countries, there is no separation based on populations, goods or providers: private insurance complements public insurance, either financially (to fund co-payments as in France) or in terms of quality of care (to buy better access, as in Ireland) (Polton and Rochaix, 2004).

In all countries, there are user charges and some healthcare expenditure that is not publicly financed. Generally, individuals with high expenditures and/or low incomes are likely to face lower co-payments. Yet out-of-pocket costs may result in financial barriers and inequity of access.

An important body of literature in health economics deals with this issue – more specifically the trade-off between the gains from insurance and the efficiency losses due to moral hazard. The debate has long been simplified, addressing two polarised situations (total insurance *versus* no insurance at all), neither of which is the common reality we face in our systems, with mixed systems of co-payments, co-insurance, exemptions etc. Thus the sensible question is what happens at the margin, as Blomqvist notes:

> For a given degree of insurance protection, would consumers be better off with a somewhat higher (or lower) degree of insurance? By extension, what is the optimal degree of insurance protection?
>
> (Blomqvist, 2001)

The question of moral hazard cannot be avoided. The fact that the patient (with the physician as agent) bears none of the financial cost may lead to over-consumption, and empirical research supports this. For example, a recent analysis of Swiss insurance plans showed that evidence of higher expenditures by enrolees with low deductibles is explained by selection effects (they are sicker), but also by incentive effects (over-consumption). The selection effect is, however, dominant, explaining 75% of the difference (Gardiol *et al.*, 2006). Research developments in this field are welcome, if we want to challenge the widespread idea that individual responsibility is the panacea.

Even if there are efficiency losses due to moral hazard and non-beneficial consumption, one can argue that the best way to remove inefficiencies is to promote evidence-based medicine. Also, a degree of inefficiency may be an acceptable price to pay to preserve equity: thus a totally egalitarian, totally publicly financed system would arguably still be preferable. But an evolution towards such an ideal seems unlikely, given the difficulties faced by all systems and the tensions between the pressures on expenditures and the scarcity of resources. So we are faced with the practical question: are there mixes which are better than others? How should the balance be struck between public insurance and private financing? High coverage for some services, which are free to all at the point of consumption, and no coverage for other services, as in Canada? Co-payments spread on all healthcare consumption as in France?* Partial coverage or no coverage of minor risks (such as deductibles, over-the-counter drugs)? What mechanisms best preserve equity? Ceilings (Scandinavia)? Exemption for people on low income or with serious illness (France)?

Even if we struggle to keep the principle of a publicly financed universal health insurance, we cannot avoid these issues which are currently faced by

* In these two countries, the proportion of public financing in total healthcare expenditure is similar (76% in France, 70% in Canada, according to the Organisation for Economic Co-operation and development (OECD)), but the distribution is very different: in Canada, public coverage accounts for 98% of spend on physicians' services, but only 38% of drugs; in France, the figures are 74% and 67% respectively.

decision makers. And the input that economists can give, through scientific evidence and empirical research, is valuable in a public debate which is again often dominated by ideology.

Inefficiencies on the supply side: how should these be tackled in practice?

The core idea developed by Alan Maynard is that instead of focusing on demand and funding, the priority should be to tackle supply-side inefficiencies.

Variations in clinical practice are well documented. Since the seminal paper by John Wennberg and Alan Gittelson more than 30 years ago, demonstrations have accumulated of wide variations in utilisation of services, not explained by illness, patient preference or evidence-based medicine (Wennberg and Gittelson, 1973). Despite the fact that healthcare professionals share the same body of knowledge, similar patients are treated differently.

The refinement of information systems in the healthcare field has allowed ever more detailed analysis of these variations in professional practices, in numerous fields and various countries. They have also shown that there is often a gap between actual care and practice guidelines, which can result in both over- and under-consumption. The Rand study concluding that 55% of chronically ill American adults had appropriate care has been highly publicised (McGlynn *et al.*, 2003) but there are similar studies in other countries. In France, in 2000, one diabetic patient out of four had an annual eye examination and six out of ten had the recommended laboratory test every six months (Caisse Nationale d'Assurance Maladie, 2002). The appropriateness of care can be also assessed through outcomes: in Canada, a study performed on a range of elective surgical procedures found that in 2% to 26% of the procedures, there was either no change or a deterioration of the outcomes reported by patients, with the highest percentage for cataract surgery (Wright *et al.*, 2002).

This growing body of evidence unambiguously shows that there is an important potential for quality and efficiency gains in all our healthcare systems. But the major issue is to mobilise these efficiency gains.

Progress has been made. There has been an important effort to gather and synthesise evidence, through the Cochrane collaboration and other initiatives. Agencies in charge of technology assessment, elaboration and dissemination of clinical guidelines, quality programmes and hospital accreditation have been implemented everywhere. Experiments and research have been conducted to test the impact of various interventions to influence professional behaviour. Strategies have been initiated in different countries on a large scale to promote evidence-based medicine.

However, this is obviously a very difficult task. The processes are slow, the improvements very gradual. The literature shows that there is no simple way to overcome the barriers to change; the strategies which prove to be the most effective – educational outreach approaches, ongoing feedback, multiple interventions – are also likely to be the most expensive ones (NHS Centre for Reviews and Dissemination, 1999). Although they can play a role, it is not clear whether organisational reforms or economic incentives would solve the problem. In that respect, it is interesting to note that health maintenance organisations (HMOs) in the US made important efficiency gains at the beginning, but typically then transferred the responsibility onto medical groups. It is also clear that the interests of governments and public agencies in that matter conflict with those of the healthcare industry – for example over the issue of reducing inappropriate drug prescribing. Thus there is clearly a gap between the growing scientific knowledge on inefficiencies or unwarranted variations in health care and the capacity to act on them.

CONCLUSION

All healthcare systems are faced with the same tensions: pressures to increase healthcare resources (with a conjunction of interests between providers and consumers who do not bear the cost of care), public finance constraints, and the necessity to maintain collective financing to ensure equitable access to care. Each system strives to achieve a specific balance among conflicting goals: high health outcomes, public expenditures control, quality and accessibility of care, equity (this balance may differ between countries, for example France's system favours freedom of choice, easy access and responsiveness over cost control).

Healthcare systems are built upon the principle of solidarity to prevent their regulation by market mechanisms, but this means that contradictions and tensions are inherent to the systems' functioning.

There is no simple solution to resolve these tensions. Choices have to be made, which should not be driven by individual consumer decisions taken under a budget constraint, but that must not ignore preferences expressed by the individuals, whether patients or citizens. Making these choices requires a quality of democratic debate, relying on evidence and scientific knowledge, but also on the expression of social values.

Being oversimplistic does not help this debate, and it is fallacious to mislead people into believing that there is one simple solution that will resolve these contradictions. Unfortunately, policy makers are often tempted by the rhetoric of *the* reform which will bring the necessary structural change and achieve a new balance for the system. Experts and commentators wanting to have a voice in the public debate tend to do the same; each has a 'magic bullet' to cure the healthcare system. Arguments are widespread internationally, but taking France as an example, three contrasting debating positions are currently adopted:

1 the growth of health expenditures is a direct result of waste and inefficient use of resources, and does not serve the well-being of the population. We could do better with the same or even fewer resources
2 the growth of health expenditures is a good thing, it is normal that the

richer a society is, the bigger the share of its income devoted to health. But public financing is necessarily limited and has to focus on an explicit range of services: beyond that private financing will have to increase
3 the growth of health expenditures is a good thing, and it is necessary to finance it publicly to maintain equity. All effective care has to be publicly funded.

Each of these convictions implies a different policy that decision makers supposedly avoid because they do not have the courage to confront professional lobbies (no. 1), or because they stay on archaic-minded and rigid egalitarian models (no. 2), or because they want to get rid of solidarity (no. 3). The common feature of these proposals, otherwise inspired by different ideologies in Alan Williams' classification, is that they present themselves as straightforward solutions: in that sense they do not favour the maturity of the democratic debate and the recognition that these tensions are inherent in our systems and that we will have to live with them.

REFERENCES

Barer M and Evans R (1995) Avalanche or glacier: health care and the demographic rhetoric. *Canadian Journal of Aging* **14**: 193–224.

Blomqvist A (2001) Does the economics of moral hazard need to be revisited? A comment on the paper by John Nyman. *Journal of Health Economics* **20**: 283–8.

Caisse Nationale d'Assurance Maladie (2002) Evolution de la prise en charge des diabétiques non insulino-dépendants traités entre 1998 et 2000. Paris: CNAMTS. www.ameli.fr/fileadmin/user_upload/documents/Prise_en_charge_des_diabetiques_1998_et_2000.pdf

Dormont B, Grignon M and Huber H (2006) Health expenditure growth: reassessing the threat of ageing. *Health Economics* **15**: 947–63.

Gardiol L, Geoffard PY and Grandchamp C (2006) Selection and incentive effects: an econometric study of Swiss health insurance claims data. In: Chiappori PA and Gollier C (eds) *Competitive Failures in Insurance Markets: theory and policy implications.* Cambridge, MA: MIT Press, pp. 81–96.

Gerdtham UG and Jönsson B (2000) International comparison of health expenditure. In: Culyer AJ and Newhouse JP (eds) *Handbook of Health Economics*. Amsterdam: Elsevier, pp. 11–53.

Le Cercle des Economistes (2004) Economie de la santé: une réforme? Non, une révolution. *Les Cahiers* **6**: 1–170.

Maarse H and Paulus A (2003) Has solidarity survived? A comparative analysis of the effect of social health insurance reform in four European countries. *Journal of Health Politics, Policy and Law* **28**: 585–614.

McGlynn EA, Asch SM, Adams J *et al.* (2003) The quality of health care delivered to adults in the United States. *New England Journal of Medicine* **348**(26): 2635–45.

NHS Centre for Reviews and Dissemination (1999) Getting evidence into practice. *Effective Health Care* **5**: 1–16.

Polton D (2004) La concurrence par le financement fonctionne-t-elle? L'expérience des HMO aux USA. *Revue d'Économie Financière* **76**: 69–85.

Polton D and Rochaix L (2004) Partage optimal entre assurance maladie privée et publique: la situation Française au regard d'expériences étrangères. *Economie Publique* **14**: 7–23.

Rice T (1998) *The Economics of Health Reconsidered.* Chicago: Health Administration Press.

Wennberg J and Gittelson A (1973) Small area variations in health care delivery: a population-based health information system can guide planning and regulatory decision-making. *Science* **182**: 1102–7.

Williams A (1988) Priority setting in public and private health care: a guide through the ideological jungle. *Journal of Health Economics* 7: 173–83.

Williams A (1974) 'Need' as a demand concept (with special reference to health). In: Culyer AJ (ed.) *Economic Policies and Social Goals. Aspects of public choice.* London: Martin Robertson, pp. 60–76.

Wright C, Chambers G K and Robens-Paradise Y (2002) Evaluation of indications for and outcomes of elective surgery. *Canadian Medical Association Journal*, **167**: 461–6.

CHAPTER 6

Resource allocation in health care: Alan Williams' decision maker, the authority and Pareto

... Anthony J Culyer

INTRODUCTION

Although this chapter is inspired overwhelmingly by the thoughts of Alan Williams, I shall begin with an aphorism of his and my long-time York colleague, Jack Wiseman:

> What is the question?' – THAT is the answer!

I shall ask some questions and try to clarify what seem to me to be some critical issues, without suggesting definitive answers. The questions are not new. I hope that my structured approach to them provides new insights. The quotation from Jack Wiseman is intended to highlight the point that answers always depend on the perspective of the questioner and the context in which the question is asked. Getting the question right is therefore a vital preliminary. Alan was, of course, very clear on his (extra-welfarist) perspective. I want to clarify what we know (believe?) and don't know about the benefits of approaching questions of resource allocation in health from a welfarist or extra-welfarist perspective. In particular, what is the difference between them?

HOW OUGHT RESOURCES TO BE ALLOCATED IN HEALTH CARE?

I shall set aside the related question of how resources ought to be allocated *to* health care and focus on the 'within health care' question. There have been two broad ways in which economists have thought about this question.

These determine, though by no means completely, the inferences that may be drawn about the effectiveness of markets as means of allocating resources to provide services; the services made available to the clients of the system; and the way in which one interprets the results of cost-effectiveness and related evaluative studies or stipulates how such studies ought to be conducted. The two approaches were first outlined by Sugden and Williams (1978) and can be characterised as 'Pareto versus the decision maker'.

THE PARETIAN APPROACH: WELFARISM, PREFERENCES AND UTILITY

In the standard welfare economics ('welfarist') approach to cost-effectiveness analysis (CEA), the general objective of expected utility maximisation is usually asserted, the value content of policy is taken to be preference based (and only preference based), the criterion for a social improvement is the Pareto (or potential Pareto) improvement, and the role of the economist is essentially that of advising those responsible for policy as to how best to improve existing resource allocations in the face of a variety of market and governmental failures. This approach to CEA ties the practice of health economics firmly into the mainstream of welfare economics, and thereby gives us handles for discriminating between 'good' and 'bad' examples of the art as practised in the literature. It also provides some intellectual underpinnings for a fairly rarefied form of libertarian politics, and it seems to be the approach adopted by at least half of the world's academic health economists.

It was not, however, the approach favoured by Alan Williams. He was more pragmatic, although as adept as any at generating elegant analyses and proofs, and at posing and solving brainteasers. He was also, incidentally, an unusually adept virtuoso – in the Harry Johnson class – at three-dimensional geometry (witness Williams, 1963).

THE DECISION-MAKER APPROACH: EXTRA-WELFARISM

The other approach is pragmatic ('extra-welfarist') as per Alan Williams, and somewhat *ad hoc*. It too begins with primitive axioms, but these are not of the formal kind that constitute the elementary propositions upon which the edifice of welfare economics is built. The most basic of these is an assumption that it is *someone other than the economist* who possesses ethical authority (usually through a political process, such as popular democracy, recognised by the analyst to be a legitimate process) to stipulate the objective of any system, of which the healthcare system in a jurisdiction is but one. This is the person designated in Sugden and Williams (1978) as 'the decision maker'. This is by far the most signal difference between the two approaches in analytical terms, since beyond this point the analysis – about maximisation of a function subject to resource constraints – is at the broadest level the same. Thus, to take again a common pursuit of health economists and again one for which Alan Williams was famous (e.g. Williams, 1981, 1983, 1985, 1986, 1988a, 1988b, 1991a, 1991b, 1992, 1993a, 1993b, 1994, 1998a, 1998b) if 'health' or 'health gain' maximisation is delivered to the economist *qua* analyst as 'the' objective of a healthcare system, then the analyst seeks the first-order maximising conditions for this under a resource constraint and sets about advising those responsible for policy as to how best to improve existing resource allocations in the face of a variety of market and governmental failures.

This approach is inherently less stable. Its foundation rests upon an external source like 'a minister' which is itself inherently unstable. It raises different brainteasers, for example, from those that arise from the probability that different 'ministers' will have different and mutually conflicting objectives measured, moreover, by quite different metrics. These objectives may make quite different claims upon our consciences. This approach raises its own interesting puzzles, such as the construct validity of 'health' and the adequacy of empirical approximations to it, the extent to which preferences (whose?) count at all in practical analyses, or how opportunity cost is assessed (are healthcare costs to be evaluated with respect to resources it uses outside the healthcare sector?) This in turn raises questions about how the efficiency of other sectors, with which health care competes for resources, should be appraised, their outcomes compared and valued, and their budgets determined.

The extra-welfarist approach is much more likely to be attuned to the issues as seen by the ultimate clients of economic analyses. Even the language of analysis is likely to be more easily communicable to non-economists – including ministers, their agents and research collaborators from other disciplines. It also has the characteristic of modesty. One might imagine it gaining Keynes' approval, for

> If economists could manage to get themselves thought of as humble, competent people, on a level with dentists, that would be splendid!
>
> (Keynes, 1931, p. 373)

SOME ROOTS OF EXTRA-WELFARISM

Several ideas provide the seeds from which extra-welfarism has grown. One was sown by Tobin (1970). He argued that the desire for equality is specific rather than general (coining the term 'specific egalitarianism'). Some basic goods and services (like health care) are, as a matter of empirical fact, commonly thought to be more properly allocated in egalitarian ways. Similar ideas are met in other disciplines. The philosopher Rawls (1971) used the notion of 'basic goods', although he explicitly excluded both health and health care from his list of 'primary goods'. The early development of health economics involved much discussion about the extent to which health care was 'different' from other goods and services: the consensus seemed to be that 'health' and health care are subject to so many of the standard cautions against reliance on free market methods of production and distribution that they are, indeed, different – partly because each specific feature looms large (severe information asymmetry, imperfect agency, inherent monopoly, absence of prices for all entities, incompleteness of markets, moral hazard, adverse selection, externality, equity), and partly because few other goods and services, if any, provide so comprehensive a challenge to efficiency and equity in resource allocation.

A second seed was sown in the shape of 'merit goods' (Musgrave, 1959): goods that need not be public goods but that are deemed so 'meritorious' that they ought to be publicly subsidised – though what qualified such goods as 'meritorious' was never quite clear, in particular it was never clear how these goods differed from goods whose consumption generated externalities (Culyer, 1971).

A third, especially influential, seed was sown by Sen (1979, 1980, 1985) in arguing that a welfarist focus on utility was too narrow. It ought to be replaced by a broader perspective that took account of the *quality* of utility and focused on people's *capabilities* rather than sensations, that is the emotional reaction (i.e. utility) of individuals to the possession of goods.

A fourth seed is the apparently explicit rejection of strict welfarist values by governments. In the UK, for example, we have on ministerial authority that health maximisation, not welfare maximisation, is the objective of the health services: 'The purpose of the NHS is to secure through the resources available the greatest possible improvement in the physical and mental health of the people of England [and] . . . aims to judge its results under three headings: equity, efficiency, and responsiveness' (Department of Health, 1996). Nothing explicit about utility or willingness to pay there!

A fifth significant seed was the 'decision-making' approach to cost–benefit analysis suggested by Sugden and Williams (1978). They contrasted the Paretian welfarist approach with its embodiment of 'individual sovereignty' with one in which 'decision makers' were the source of values (and weights) in public decision making.

Underlying these extra-welfarist views are two disturbing questions for economists. One is this: granted that people have knowable preferences, what is the link between the satisfaction of these preferences and welfare? Is there, indeed, any link? If there is, how many ways are there of describing the various psychological states that might constitute welfare? Moreover, does not the quality of a preference matter – like whether it is a preference for something good or something evil, cheap or superficial, noble or profound? The other disturbing question comes from challenging the convention that public decision makers, as agents for the public, ought to act as they think the public (their principals) would act. Suppose instead, however, that they were to act rather as they think the principals *ought* to act? Ought decision makers to act as 'moral' agents?

PARETO VERSUS THE DECISION MAKER: SOME HEAD-TO-HEAD COMPARISONS

The standard sorts of intellectual journey that economists make here have a common root but, beyond a certain stage, diverge. I think they can best be described as a sequence that moves in steps. These are summarised in Figure 6.1 and then I discuss each step individually.

(a) Primitive proposition: 'normative economics is done to serve the social good'

↓

(b) The social good depends (only?) on characteristics of (all?) individuals, the distribution of these characteristics and (possibly) the nature of the interrelationships between individuals

↓

(c) The social good can be conceived as quantifiable, in the sense of being measurable up to a linear transformation, and as being some kind of (weighted?) sum of the things on which the social good depends (only on this?)

↓	↓
(d) Realising the social good equates to maximising welfare (satisfaction? well-being? happiness? ophelimity?)	Realising the social good equates to optimising over an eclectic set of characteristics of individuals or groups of individuals ('welfare' can be one of them, 'health' another)
↓	↓
(e) Welfare is a function (only?) of individual 'preferences' (these may be 'true', 'underlying', 'stated' . . . preferences)	The constituents of the social good are context dependent and determined by an 'ethical authority' for that context (e.g. the 'minister of health')
↓	↓
(f) The relevant preferences are (only?) those over goods and services or (possibly?) the characteristics of goods and services	While preferences may be important, other considerations (feelings? capacities? capabilities? values? interests? perceptions? relationships? processes?) may also have significance
↓	↓
(g) Preferences can be revealed (approximately) either through market transactions or through experiments	Some elements may be revealed (approximately) through transactions or experiments, others may be assessed better through other methods such as deliberation (or with a combination of methods)
↓	↓
(h) Preference equates to 'utility'	Preference-based utility is but one consideration

cont.

↓	↓
(i) Decisions can be informed by the agenda-setting/question-provoking, taxonomising methods of CEA etc	(i) Decisions can be informed by the agenda-setting/question-provoking, taxonomising methods of CEA etc
↓	↓
(j) Distributional concerns or interpersonal comparisons of welfare (utility) cannot be addressed with Paretianism	Distributional concerns or interpersonal comparisons of subjective states may be an important part of the analysis, though there is precious little guidance as to how they are to be addressed and how they are to be combined with efficiency criteria
↓	↓
(k) Public decisions can be modelled or 'made' through algorithmic processes like CEA (which may embody other algorithms, like quality-adjusted life years (QALYs))	Public decisions can be informed by algorithmic processes, but often need to be supplemented by deliberative processes that are context dependent to assist the process of conflict resolution over values, to weigh up the significance of other contributors to the social good and to carry conviction with 'the public'

FIGURE 6.1 Sequential steps in Paretian versus decision-maker approaches to public decision making

a. Primitive proposition 'normative economics is done to serve the social good'

Step (a) contains a primitive proposition of the kind of statement that does indeed underlie most of what has usually been called 'welfare economics'. It establishes a normative context for the analysis and implies the existence of an entity called 'society'. Like any such point of departure, it is taken largely uncritically. Most of the debates that take place are downstream from it.

b. The social good depends (only?) on characteristics of (all?) individuals, the distribution of these characteristics and (possibly) the nature of the interrelationships between individuals

Step (b) says what it is that the social good depends on. It is an assertion that is not necessarily entailed by step (a). The emphasis that economists typically put on the individual characteristics, their distribution across individuals, and the nature of the interrelationships between individuals (are they loving, respectful and trusting, or hate filled, inconsiderate and suspicious) varies a good deal. But what is overwhelmingly the case is that the focus is on individuals. Needless to say, the main 'characteristic' used in welfare economics is 'preference', but in step (b) the question of what the characteristics comprise is left open.

c. The social good can be conceived as quantifiable, in the sense of being measurable up to a linear transformation, and as being some kind of (weighted?) sum of the things on which the social good depends (only on this?)

Step (c) provides the means by which most economists do their work: it permits marginal analysis; it addresses the 'adding-up' problem, both of the characteristics that are asserted in step (b) for one individual and of the resultant sums across many individuals. The question 'which individuals?' is usually left unaddressed. The presumption seems to be one of inclusivity, though sometimes explicit exclusions are encountered – such as children, the crazed, the unconscious or the irrational. The latter may not necessarily correspond to those who do not obey the axioms of expected utility theory, presumably on the grounds that such an exclusion would be altogether too comprehensive for comfort, since so few people seem actually to obey those axioms (for extensive reviews of this literature, see Hogarth and Reder, 1987; Kahneman *et al.*, 1999; Kahneman and Tversky, 2000).

d. Realising the social good equates to maximising welfare (satisfaction? well-being? happiness? ophelimity?)

or / versus

Realising the social good equates to optimising over an eclectic set of characteristics of individuals or groups of individuals ('welfare' can be one of them, 'health' another)

At step (d) there is a decided branching. It relates to the character of the entities to be maximised or equitably distributed. In the left-hand column is what I understand to be the conventional route of welfare economics. This is welfarism with the social good being more precisely located in terms of the satisfaction of preferences. Welfare, well-being, satisfaction, happiness, ophelimity and so on, while not being synonyms or even plesionyms, are conceptual bed-fellows. The bed they occupy is the procrustean one of a state of mind called 'preference'. The fellows are quite diverse, united by their common respect for individual preferences (although not much else).

On the right-hand side we find a more tentative and open-ended line of enquiry. Welfare, in any of the senses on the left-hand side, counts as one – but only one – of a set of relevant characteristics of individuals or groups. Groups need to be there because of the possibility that one may wish to include some characteristics of *relationships between individuals* in the idea of the social good. In this specific sense, extra-welfarism might allow 'society' to be more than a collection of atomistic individuals. Although the right-hand side approach may entail maximising some function of these diverse entities, it may not go so far (stopping, for example, at listing and measuring the variables in question as in 'cost–consequences analysis'), or it may take a fuzzier approach ('satisficing', for example). Its eclecticism is attractive to any who want to associate the idea of the social good with human experiences and characteristics other than those normally subsumed under the heading of 'preferences'. Eclectic candidates might include ability to adapt to changing circumstances, achievements, aspirations, assurances and reassurances, being appreciated, being consulted, being free, being informed, capabilities, capacities to benefit, entering or leaving 'states of being', fearing or not fearing for the public safety of oneself or one's children, fears in general, feelings that are not preferences, participation in processes of many kinds, security, senses of belonging and self-worth, senses of membership in a kindly and mutually supportive society, virtue, and other such things. Most – probably all – can be measured, albeit with varying degrees of construct validity, in accordance with the prescriptions of step (c) but without any pretence that it is *preference* that is being measured.

The opening up of so disparate a range of considerations has important consequences. For example, following the right-hand column in a context in which 'being free' is a major element of the objective function might prove more antagonistic to government regulation and 'interference' than any such case mounted on a Paretian platform. It is likely to provoke two kinds of response from left-leaning economists (in the columnar sense). The first of these two responses is to say that the entire scheme is preposterously ambitious; far better to exercise some modesty by recognising that the economist's role is restricted to a narrower set of preference-based considerations that we may call 'economic welfare' and the rest are someone else's business. The counter to this is twofold. First, it may be – and it often actually is – business that no one else is around to pick up. Second, economists rarely hedge their advice, whether about the operation of markets in general, or of those in or connected with the healthcare sector, by disclaimers about all the possibly relevant considerations they are ignoring. The modesty, in short, is a sham and the rest of the world is invited to accept policy prescriptions that appear, at least on some occasions, as grotesque, like the appropriateness, to use Uwe Reinhardt's telling example (Reinhardt, 1998), of an idea of efficiency that has poor and sickly baby Smith consuming a small fraction of the health care consumed by rich and healthy baby Chen.

The other kind of response from the left-leaning (in the columnar sense) economist is to say that all the 'extras' that right-leaning economists want to allow, at least in principle, are as admissible on the left as they are on the right, in that there are preferences over them all – we can even have preferences over preferences – and utility numbers are readily available to be assigned to them by well-known experimental methods. There is but a short solipsistic step to the *reductio ad absurdam* of supposing that every attitude is a 'preference' and every difficult choice is a utilitarian trade-off – as though there really were no difference between the questions 'what do I, a person with preferences, *want* to do?' and 'what *ought* I to do, I, having preferences but wanting to be behave morally?' or as if there were not a possible – even frequent – conflict between the answers to these two questions. It also blithely ignores the genuine puzzle: what is so special about 'preferences' that we want to erect our idea of social welfare entirely upon them? Moreover, even if we do not go beyond preferences, we ought surely to care about their ethical character. The same kind of solipsistic thinking leads to the absurd Panglossian conclusion that all is at all times for the best in the world, otherwise it would have changed. If it didn't, then the expected utility of the world changed must have been less than the expected utility of the world kept constant; the gainers evidently could not compensate the losers. And the costs of reducing the transaction costs that may have impeded some transactions must have been higher than the combined surplus to be had from making the transactions that were not made – otherwise those costs would have been incurred and the transactions thus enabled would have been executed (Culyer, 1984).

A clear danger in the right-hand column arises from the risk of double-counting or over- and under-accounting. Whereas there are standard procedures for avoiding these biasing distortions in conventional welfare economics – transfers and sunk costs are not confused with opportunity costs; increased property values are not added to the value of shortened commuting times – the opportunities for missing such effects on the right is much enhanced by the plethora of possible elements. Avoidance requires clarity about the elements and an understanding of how they may be empirically related.

Step (d) is the point at which there seems to be a clear separation of 'welfarism' and 'extra-welfarism'. I am using the term 'extra-welfarism' throughout in order to differentiate it from a more extreme 'non-welfarism' (Kaplow and Shavell, 2001; Dolan and Olsen, 2002) which appears to deny the relevance of any part of the welfarist programme (and preferences in particular) in helping to identify the social good.

e. Welfare is a function (only?) of individual 'preferences' (these may be 'true', 'underlying', 'stated'... preferences)

or / versus

The constituents of the social good are context-dependent and determined by an 'ethical authority' for that context (e.g. the 'minister of health')

In step (e) we explicitly lay bare the roots of welfarism in preference relations, with the tentative suggestion that welfare is dependent only on the satisfaction of preferences, with some acknowledgment of the fact that 'preferences' are not self-evident and generally have to be inferred via fairly precarious chains of reasoning from behaviours of one kind or another. The basis of welfare in preferences is, however, essentially stipulative and *a priori*. It is therefore a serious embarrassment to be told, as we increasingly are, that the measurement of preference is an empirical will-o'-the-wisp (Kelman, 2005). On the right-hand side we may still retain welfare (despite doubts) in the preferential sense, but its retention is conditional on the nature and circumstances of the decisions to be made. The ethical authority comes not from a stipulative condition about what welfare is, but from an ethical arbiter – or a process through which such an arbiter is to be identified. In the one case, the ethics come from the characteristics of the axioms, including their factual truth; in the other from the legitimacy of the arbiter – such as whether she has been elected. Essentially, the right-hand side substitutes a process (a stipulator or a method of finding one) for an algorithm.

f. The relevant preferences are (only?) those over goods and services or (possibly?) the characteristics of goods and services

or / versus

While preferences may be important, other considerations (feelings? capacities? capabilities? values? interests? perceptions? relationships? processes?) may also have significance

The left-hand side of step (f) has two variants: preferences are considered to be either over goods and services or over characteristics of goods and services (examples might be their effectiveness, convenience and responsiveness). On the right-hand side such preferences may also be important, but other factors may also be deemed relevant such as the employment conditions of those delivering the services or whether the service delivery team treats patients as partners in a treatment and rehabilitation process. Some utilitarians on the left include 'process' in principle and that is a somewhat less restrictive form of welfarism than that delineated in the table.

g. Preferences can be revealed (approximately) either through market transactions or through experiments

or / versus

Some elements may be revealed (approximately) through transactions or experiments, others may be assessed better through other methods such as deliberation (or with a combination of methods)

Step (g) concerns the measurement of the sources of welfare. On the left, preferences may be inferred from market transactions or through experiments in either real (relative) terms or by a monetary yardstick – willingness to pay or willingness to accept. On the right, the same techniques may be applied and inferences drawn for preferences deemed relevant; some of them may also prove suitable for measuring and valuing non-preference elements (for example, limits placed on the application of the 'rule of rescue' or the discovery of distributional weights from economic experiments); but there will often be other considerations that may require altogether different mechanisms of empirical inference and appraisal through, for example, consultation and negotiation (for example, the short-term service impact of a new addition to the drug formulary on general practitioners (GPs) and pharmacies and its managerial implications; or working out in committee an agreed formula for ranking needs; or whether a proposed allocation mechanism may be seen as an embarrassing political symbol or precedent).

More fundamentally, experimental economics and psychology have revealed major ambiguities in what we may understand by 'preference'. These partly impact on the meanings one attaches to 'rationality', and partly suggest that 'real' preferences (if they can be said to exist at all) are virtually impossible to reveal. They also suggest that whatever it is that experiments and like mechanisms reveal is highly contingent on circumstances – not merely the circumstances of the birth and environment of the subject of the experiment but the immediate circumstances under which whatever is being revealed is revealed – such as framing effects and the like (Kahneman and Tversky, 2000). This opens up the tantalising possibility of systems for ordering public policy options that make no pretence at accuracy in their portrayal of preferences or people's states of mind and that might even go further and be the ranking decisions of committees based upon whatever virtues are deemed acceptable by the 'authority'. It seems an attractive quality of a public health policy mechanism that it ought to aim in some way to reflect what seem to be the values of stakeholders (especially the general public and those most directly affected by health care – patients and their families), for which decision makers would be accountable, and which would resemble utilities in their form and structure but would not necessarily be seeking to represent 'preferences'. The challenge is to decide whether welfarism or extra-welfarism is better able to embody such values.

h. Preference equates to 'utility'

or / versus

Preference-based utility is but one consideration

Step (h) contains several causes of potential confusion. Because of the greater inclusivity of the right-hand column, the utility measures appropriate to the left-hand column may also be relevant on the right. Moreover, one can also have utility measures of non-preference entities and, when this is the case, the differences between the two columns become blurred. The problem here is that 'utility' is doing more work than it can normally bear. For example, in addressing the matter of health outcomes one might:

- ask the following types of people to assign utility numbers according to a conventional experimental method to states of health-related quality life:
  - — doctors
  - — patients with the specified condition
  - — all patients
  - — taxpayers
  - — informal carers
- where the subjects may be members of the class described and asked to assign their own values or be non-members but asked to assign numbers

putting themselves in the shoes of those indicated (revealing something resembling the 'ethical preferences' of Harsanyi (1955)). In either case the experiment is designed to measure preferences

- assign utility numbers in the foregoing experiment and its variants according to the subjects' view of:
  — the desert of the probable beneficiaries
  — the productivity of the probable beneficiaries
  — the likely income generated for the service providers.

In each of these cases, the term 'utility' may be entirely appropriate in, say, the conventional sense of being normative and requiring ordering systems to be used that are characterised by completeness, transitivity, continuity, convexity and non-satiation. But the normative significance is quite different according to who is doing the assigning, whose utility is being measured – if anyone's – and according to whether utility is being used as an index of preference, or health, or need, or of some other desideratum that enables decision makers to prioritise uses for resources.

i. Decisions can be informed by the agenda-setting/question-provoking, taxonomising methods of CEA etc

Step (i) identifies an underrated virtue of economics, which is its taxonomising capability – the categorisation of elements for a decision maker to consider. These might include the critical significance of 'perspective', the sources of bias in signals about values and what can be done about them, the range of possible consequences, external effects, publicness of goods and bads, the insights to be had from sensitivity analyses, the distinction between (and therefore searching testing of) elements claimed to be 'fixed' rather than 'variable', the idea of opportunity cost and its meaning in the presence and absence of market signals, the idea that speed of implementation is a determinant of cost, and so on. This agenda-setting feature appears in both columns. Since the right-hand column is the more inclusive column, it must imply that some of the elements in a choice that may be thrown up in an initial brainstorming session using an economic 'checklist' would be deemed 'beyond' the scope of an economic analysis that was to be conducted according to the rules of the left-hand column.

j. Distributional concerns or interpersonal comparisons of welfare (utility) cannot be addressed with Paretianism

or / versus

Distributional concerns or interpersonal comparisons of subjective states may be an important part of the analysis, though there is precious little guidance as to how they are to be addressed and how combined with efficiency criteria

Step (j) is not really a step in the Paretian scheme at all, since interpersonal comparisons of subjective experiences, such as 'welfare' or 'utility', are either excluded by design or surreptitiously sneaked in by less careful analysts. Some have explicitly urged the use of unitary weights (e.g. Harberger's third postulate in Harberger (1971)). Alan Williams himself urged the use of a system of weighting that discriminated against older people (Williams, 1997, 1998b). The approach adopted to date by others on the right is scarcely more advanced however. Harberger (1978) explicitly analysed the qualitative effects of differential weights in the use of consumers' and producers' surplus in cost–benefit analysis, though – unlike Williams – without analysis of the source and moral authority of such weights. Advice from, for example, the National Institute for Health and Clinical Excellence (NICE) includes: treating unitary weights as provisional, conducting sensitivity analyses to test the impact of alternative weights on the application of a decision rule, taking account of the views of advisory bodies on specific distributional questions, conducting research into the distributional values that are held by the public, and embodying these concerns in the deliberative processes that translate economic and other evidence into practical advice for policy and professional practice, rather than embodying them in the economic evidence itself (NICE, 2004).

k. Public decisions can be modelled or 'made' through algorithmic processes like CEA (which may embody other algorithms, like QALYs)

or / versus

Public decisions can be informed by algorithmic processes, but often need to be supplemented by deliberative processes that are context dependent to assist the process of conflict resolution over values, to weigh up the significance of other contributors to the social good and to carry conviction with 'the public'

Step (k) contains a more striking contrast between the two columns and develops the point just made about process. I may have overdrawn the distinction, but I think it is a real one which accords to the left-hand column a more 'deterministic' form of analysis than in the right-hand column. Both employ algorithms and models, but the right-hand column emphasises that at least parts of the agenda may be best addressed through a deliberative process. This is not quite the same as a consultative process. Through consultative processes one can gain information, even scientific information (if the consulting is done in a scientific way, for example by commissioning economists to discover people's willingnesses to pay for additional QALYs), but the final decision is bound to be determined by the combining of what Lomas and colleagues (2005) call context-free scientific evidence, context-sensitive scientific evidence and colloquial evidence. The difference between the first two of these is well illustrated by the difference between explanatory and pragmatic trials, the former being rather good (one hopes) at establishing internal validity, and the latter (again, one hopes) at establishing external validity. Colloquial evidence is not scientific evidence at all, though frequently it is the only form of evidence available to a decision maker. It typically consists of 'case studies', guesses about what the political and other constraints on the scope of a decision may be, 'expert opinion' (which may be scientifically collected but which is still a species of gossip – systematically collected gossip). Weighing all these matters up is, I conjecture, better done through a deliberative process involving the relevant 'stakeholders'. I also conjecture that considering matters of equity is also most fruitfully done in a deliberative fashion, especially if controversial. To the extent that this is true, economists become much more intimately involved in – and responsible for – public policy resource allocation decisions. The phenomenon is well illustrated by the way in which NICE's appraisal committees work.

A QUESTION OF AUTHORITY

One way of interpreting the distinction between the left and the right columns is through an idea of 'authority'. On the left the moral authority underlying 'ought' statements of public policy comes to us *a priori*, as in ethics – in this case preference utilitarianism. On the right, the ethical authority underlying 'ought' statements is *ad hoc*; it is externally provided, typically for most practical purposes, by a senior accountable politician having formal responsibility for a sphere of policy. This comes close to Alan Williams' claim that CEA and related techniques were 'value-free presupposing no ethical principles at all' (Sugden and Williams, 1978, p. 235). The main case against the left-hand column view is that it excludes too many considerations that may be relevant in decision contexts in the sphere of social policy. The main case against the right-hand view is that it might be used to exclude the appropriate use of the left, for it would be foolish to deny the possibility that Paretianism, perhaps with a well-judged dash of adjusted 'Harbergerism' in the matter of weights, may on occasion be all that is required. However, the 'adjustment' I have in mind is one that generates non-arbitrary interpersonal weights, which might be, but is unlikely to be, unitary. Unfortunately, the source for such weights plainly cannot be the economist *qua* economist and must surely be the 'authority'.

VALUES, PREFERENCES AND DECISION PROCESSES

I have suggested that a deliberative process may be the natural decision-making process to accompany a right-handed view of the use of economic evaluation in resource allocation decisions. Whether that is so will plainly depend in part on the range and character of the elements of analysis that transcend standard welfarism. It will also depend on the context of the decision (for example, whether it is one to be made on behalf of whole populations or major subgroups of populations as distinct from made in a one-to-one situation between the professional and patient). Finally, the value of using deliberative processes will also depend on much broader social and political considerations – concepts of respect for the individual, agency, paternalism and the like.

It seems axiomatic that no method of making choices can long survive – nor ought it – if it is divorced from the values of the people it is there to serve. This is as true of methods that serve the interests of dominant elites as it is of those that serve the interests of entire populations. A challenge arises from the need to encompass different cultures and values – and even preferences. Another comes from the need for the processes *to be seen* to be encompassing different cultures and so on. Constrained outcomes, no matter how satisfactory, are never going to be believed to have been truly the best that could have been achieved if they are generated by processes that are secret. Yet another comes from the fact (conjecture?) that people are much more likely to believe in the authenticity of a decision if they, or those whom they trust, have participated in the making of it. Indeed, this is one of the attractions of the perfect market model – no transaction takes place without the active consent of any affected parties (assuming of course that there are exchangeable and enforceable private property rights in everything), so no values are crowded out (not even the famous transactions of Sen's sadist and masochist), the outcome is as visible as the participants wish it to be, and everyone who needs to be involved is involved.

SOME QUESTIONS TO WHICH I DO NOT KNOW THE ANSWERS

Let me end by proposing some further questions without attempting to answer them.

- Is it possible to make general statements about the character of decisions that determine the balance of algorithmic and deliberative resolution of value questions?
- Is it desirable, supposing it to be possible, to retain any element of preference-based welfarism in cost-effectiveness and related techniques of analysis as applied in health care?
- Where it is decided to go beyond, or simply to circumnavigate, preferences (one might say 'extra-preferentially'), what kinds of ethical authority ought we to seek?
- How are controversies over interpersonal weights to be resolved and any such resolution embodied in economic analyses?
- Without a foundation of 'preferences' what roles are there for 'utility'?
- What kind of accountability to the general public is required?
- Supposing that we also want (or are instructed by 'the authority') to keep public policy in line with common values in society, how best do we do this (invite comments, use consultation, citizens' juries, markets or pseudo-markets . . .?)

'What is the question?' – THAT is the answer!

REFERENCES

Culyer AJ (1971) Merit goods and the welfare economics of coercion. *Public Finance* **26**: 546–72.

Culyer AJ (1984) The quest for efficiency in the public sector: economists versus Dr Pangloss (or why conservative economists are not nearly conservative enough). In: Hanusch H (ed.) *Public Finance and the Quest for Efficiency*. Proceedings of the 38th Congress of the UPF, Copenhagen, Detroit: Wayne State University Press, pp. 39–48.

Department of Health (1996) *Priorities and Planning Guidance for the NHS 1997/98*. London: Department of Health.

Dolan P and Olsen JA (2002) *Distributing Health Care: economic and ethical issues*. Oxford: Oxford University Press.

Harberger AC (1971) Three basic postulates for applied welfare economics: an interpretive essay. *Journal of Economic Literature* **9**: 785–97.

Harberger AC (1978) On the use of distributional weights in social cost-benefit analysis, *Journal of Political Economy* **86**: S87–S120.

Harsanyi J (1955) Cardinal welfare, individualistic ethics and interpersonal comparisons of utility. *Journal of Political Economy* **63**: 309–21.

Hogarth R and Reder M (eds) (1987) *Rational Choice: the contrast between economics and psychology*. Chicago: University of Chicago Press.

Kahneman D, Diener E and Schwarz N (eds) (1999) *Well-Being: the foundations of hedonic psychology*. New York: Russell Sage Foundation.

Kahneman D and Tversky A (eds) (2000) *Choice, Values and Frames*. Cambridge: Cambridge University Press.

Kaplow L and Shavell S (2001) Any non-welfarist method of policy assessment violates the Pareto principle. *Journal of Political Economy* **109**: 281–6.

Kelman M (2005) Hedonic psychology and the ambiguities of 'welfare'. *Philosophy and Public Affairs* **33**: 391–412.

Keynes JM (1931) *Essays in Persuasion*. London: Macmillan.

Lomas J, Culyer AJ, McCutcheon C, McAuley L and Law S (2005) *Conceptualizing and Combining Evidence for Health System Guidance*. Ottawa: Canadian Health Services Research Foundation.

Musgrave RA (1959) *The Economics of Public Finance*. New York: McGraw Hill.

National Institute for Clinical Excellence (2004) *Guide to the Methods of Technology Appraisal* (ref. N0515). Available at: www.nice.org.uk/page.aspx?o=201973

Rawls J (1971) *A Theory of Justice*. Cambridge MA: Harvard University Press.

Reinhardt U (1998) Abstracting from distributional effects, this policy is efficient. In: Barer ML, Getzen TE and Stoddart GL (eds) *Health, Health Care and Health Economics, Perspectives on Distribution*. New York: John Wiley and Sons, pp. 1–52.

Sen AK (1979) Personal utilities and public judgments: or what's wrong with welfare economics. *Economic Journal* **589**: 537–8.

Sen AK (1980) *Equality of What? The Tanner lectures on human values*. Cambridge: Cambridge: Cambridge University Press.

Sen AK (1985) *Commodities and Capabilities*. Amsterdam: North Holland.

Sugden R and Williams A (1978) *The Principles of Practical Cost–Benefit Analysis*. New York, Oxford: Oxford University Press.

Tobin J (1970) On limiting the domain of inequality. *Journal of Law and Economics* **13**: 263–77.

Williams A (1963) *Public Finance and Budgetary Policy*. London: Allen and Unwin.

Williams A (1981) Welfare economics and health status measurement. In: Van der Gaag J and Perlman M (eds) *Health, Economics and Health Economics*. Amsterdam: North-Holland, pp. 159–70.

Williams A (1983) The role of economics in the evaluation of health care technologies. In: Culyer AJ and Horisberger B (eds) *Economic and Medical Evaluation of Health Care Technologies: papers presented at a symposium held April 1982, Wolfsberg, Switzerland*. Berlin: Springer Verlag, pp. 38–68.

Williams A (1985) Economics of coronary artery bypass grafting. *British Medical Journal* **291**: 326–9.

Williams A (1986) Health economics: the cheerful face of the dismal science? In Williams AH (ed.) *Health and Economics: Proceedings of Section F (Economics) of the British Association for the Advancement of Science, Bristol, 1986*. Houndmills: Macmillan, pp. 1–11.

Williams A. (1988a) Priority setting in public and private health care: a guide through the ideological jungle, *Journal of Health Economics*, 7, 173–183.

Williams A (1988b) Ethics and efficiency in the provision of health care. In: Bell JM and Mendus S (eds) *Philosophy and Medical Welfare*. (Royal Institute of Philosophy Lecture Series 23, Supplement to Philosophy). Cambridge: Cambridge University Press, pp. 111–26.

Williams A (1991a) Some methodological issues in the use of cost-benefit analysis in health care. *Osaka Economic Papers* **40**: 63–9.

Williams A (1991b) Is the QALY a technical solution to a political problem? Of course not! *International Journal of Health Services* **21**: 365–9.

Williams A (1992) Cost-effectiveness analysis: is it ethical? *Journal of Medical Ethics* **18**: 7–11.

Williams A (1993a) Cost-benefit analysis: applied welfare economics or general decision aid. In: Williams A and Giardina E (eds) *Efficiency in the Public Sector*. Aldershot: Edward Elgar, pp. 65–79.

Williams A (1993b) Some methodological issues in the use of cost-benefit analysis in health care. In El-Agraa AM (ed.) *Public and International Economics*. New York: St Martin's Press, pp. 33–4.

Williams A (1994) Economics, society and health care ethics. In: Gillon R (ed.) *Principles of Health Care Ethics*. Chichester: John Wiley and Sons, pp. 829–42.

Williams A (1997) Intergenerational equity: an exploration of the 'fair innings' argument. *Health Economics* **6**: 117–32.

Williams A (1998a) QALYs and ethics: a health economist's perspective. *Social Science and Medicine* **43**: 1795–804.

Williams A (1998b) If we are going to get a fair innings, someone will need to keep the score! In: Barer M and Stoddart G (eds) *Health, Health Care and Health Economics: perspectives on distribution*. Chichester: John Wiley and Son, pp. 319–30.

CHAPTER 7

Discussion of Anthony Culyer's paper: 'Resource allocation in health care: Alan Williams' decision maker, the authority, and Pareto'

... Adrian Towse

Tony's paper is intended to take us to a better understanding of the relevance of welfarist and extra-welfarist approaches to rationing the provision of health care. I follow Tony in also characterising these approaches as the Paretian and decision-maker approaches respectively.

In making the statement 'What is the question?' – THAT is the answer!', Tony suggests that the choice of approach to address a rationing issue depends on what question we are trying to answer (and from what perspective). I agree and return to this later.

My starting point is that Tony (like most extra-welfarists) is not opposed in principle to using markets or indeed to welfarist analysis in general. He argues, rather, that an extra-welfarist approach is more comprehensive because preferences and utility are considered alongside other factors that impact on well-being, and distributional issues can also be addressed. This comprehensiveness is particularly relevant to health care, because health is a 'different' element of well-being. Hence he prefers to address healthcare rationing issues using an extra-welfarist approach.

He has three main criticisms of welfarism as an approach to resource allocation in health:

1 the focus on individual utility derived from preferences over goods and services gives a very narrow view of what matters to people. In health care it is ability to function and psychic state (which contribute to health status) and the length of life that matter. The welfarist toolkit is not helpful in this context
2 the application of willingness to pay techniques – arguably the only part of

the welfarist toolkit that is relevant to obtaining an understanding as to the values individuals put on health or other outcomes provided by the delivery of health care – is of limited value. This is because preferences have to be backed by income to count, and because the technique cannot value 'non-preference elements' such as the rule of rescue. The requirement for income to enter the equation raises major equity issues in using this approach in health care

3 the use in the standard welfarist approach of a requirement for Paretian improvement (or indeed a Kaldor–Hicks improvement) with no interpersonal comparison of utility, or even a requirement for gainers to compensate losers, makes it very restrictive. Interpersonal comparisons are essential for decision making about resource allocation in health care.

By contrast, extra-welfarism is pragmatic in several important respects:

1 the economist can focus on the objectives of the decision maker. There is no mystery as to where the objective function comes from. It is imposed. It is not the task of the economist to derive it from individual preferences (or indeed to fail as Arrow's Impossibility Theorem tells us)
2 the decision maker can have all sorts of interesting things in their objective function – they don't have to be based on, or limited to, individual utilities derived from preferences over goods and services. This, in principle, enables extra-welfarism to provide a more comprehensive view of well-being
3 economists can find innovative (and eclectic) ways of measuring the impact of interventions on the objective function, enabling the decision maker to understand whether (say) action A or action B will better help achieve their objective given a resource constraint
4 decision making can be informed by results of deliberative mechanisms, i.e. individuals discussing issues and collectively reaching a view as to their preferences between social outcomes (e.g. which groups of patients should get access to treatment).

This contrast gives rise to a number of questions which I consider briefly in the rest of my paper:

1 which is the more useful 'general theory' of resource allocation?
2 is health special?
3 what is the role for preference elicitation in extra-welfarism?
4 is extra-welfarism as pragmatic and eclectic as implied – and indeed welfarism as incomplete?
5 does welfarism have nothing to offer on distributional matters?
6 is there a role for welfarism in healthcare resource allocation?

WHICH IS THE 'GENERAL THEORY?'

In step (f), Tony sets out the limitations of the welfarist reliance on preferences over goods and services. To paraphrase, humankind cannot live by preferences alone – to focus on goods and services is 'commodity fetishism'. It is helpful to draw on Sen's framework for thinking about well-being (or, in Sen's terms, the 'standard of living') (Sen, 1987a, 1987b). This is summarised in Figure 7.1.

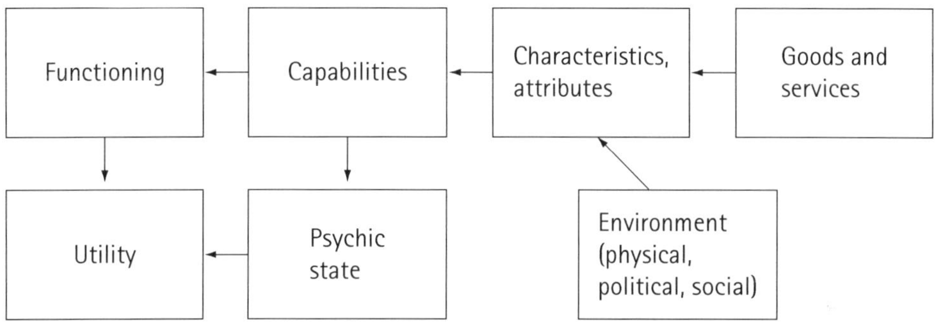

FIGURE 7.1 Utilities, functionings, capabilities and their sources. Adapted from Muellbauer J (1987) Professor Sen on the Standard of Living. In: Hawthorn G (ed.) *The Standard of Living*. Cambridge: Cambridge University Press. Used and adapted with permission of Cambridge University Press.

What really determines peoples' well-being is their capabilities, functioning and psychic state. Goods and services play an important part of this. But so do many other things including their physical environment and their social and family relationships. The extra-welfarist framework is helpful in addressing public policy issues, including the measurement of 'national income' and resource allocation in public services such as health care. But it is not clear that its all-embracing nature offers any conceptual or practical advantages in analysing markets for most goods and services. As Tony recognises, welfarists might argue that theirs is the general theory and that the utility framework can deal with these other factors – for example, individuals derive utility from the environment (indeed the welfarist approach of contingent valuation has played a major role in the development of environmental economics to support policy making (e.g. Arrow *et al.*, 1993)). But when we apply this to (say) family relationships Tony is right to suggest that we are better off looking at the direct benefits that people derive. Moreover, it remains unclear whether welfarism can address equity issues (see below). Neither welfarism nor extra-welfarism can therefore be seen as an approach that is universally helpful. It is clear, however, that for most goods and services the welfarist approach suffices and provides powerful analytical tools. For some key social goods (I would include health, education and justice) we are more interested in the impact on people's functioning and well-being. Society prefers to make these goods directly accessible rather than provide income and let individuals decide for themselves whether to consume them. Here extra-welfarism is more helpful. Many 'non-market' activities (including social and personal relationships) may also fit better within this approach.

IS HEALTH SPECIAL?

Health is clearly special in two senses:

- there is a lot of uncertainty in the market as well as market failure on both the demand and supply sides of the market (e.g. imperfect agency, information asymmetry and suppliers with market power). There is also strong societal concern about the impact of income inequalities on access to health care. None of these issues is unique to health care, but the combination is unusual (indeed health care may be one of the few markets where all of the standard concerns about the ability of a market to allocate efficiently may apply) and has led to substantial government intervention in the regulation, funding and supply of health care
- health is fundamental to human well-being and so access to healthcare is an essential good. It fits the Sen model. We are interested in physical functioning and psychic state. And we want to provide access to services that will improve physical and mental health – not to provide people with money with which they can choose whether to buy health care or other goods and services.

Welfarism helps us understand and analyse the market failure in health care but is less useful than extra-welfarism as a framework for resource allocation, i.e. in providing tools to address concerns about access and about the impact of health care on health status.

WHAT IS THE ROLE FOR PREFERENCE ELICITATION IN EXTRA-WELFARISM?

In health care, preferences are expressed when people choose insurance policies in both private markets and social insurance systems with competing insurers; within the tax-based NHS by patients and carers when making individual treatment decisions jointly with doctors; and by choice of provider, either when choosing a GP practice or hospital (under Patient Choice). These preferences may be shaped by supply-side issues (e.g. a patient may opt for a hospital with a shorter waiting list) and therefore help determine resource allocation issues. These are not preferences that usually interest an extra-welfarist. Their concern is primarily around health gain.

The interesting issue is therefore whether valuations (of impact on individuals) in public policy making are:

- postulated by the decision maker – the *decision-making approach*. This can be benign dictatorship, although, following Sugden (*see* Chapter 2),

it makes more sense to think of decision makers as accountable to an electorate
- inferred from market behaviour (transactions) or attempts to elicit preferences (through experiments). This is the welfarist or *Paretian approach*.

There is nothing in the extra-welfarist approach to stop the decision maker being *informed* by market behaviour or attempts to elicit preferences. Indeed one might hope that in allocating healthcare resources the decision maker wants to understand the preferences of the individuals on the menu of competing combinations of services the decision maker has to choose between.

However, extra-welfarists seem to be ambiguous about the role of preference elicitation.

On the one hand they:
- strongly favour the use of health status instruments to establish the physical functioning and mental state of individuals, i.e. what can they do/feel (although we can note Sen's opposition to self-reported morbidity because – like income-based preference measures – it can be distorted by poverty (Sen, 2002))
- support the valuation of those health status measures using individual preference-elicitation instruments grounded in decision theory (irrespective of whether patients or the public are being asked to value a health state, they are being asked to answer how it impacts/would impact on them).

On the other hand, they:
- are opposed to the use of willingness-to-pay techniques, primarily because it introduces the bias of an income constraint, but also because it moves away from measuring health towards measuring utility. Many extra-welfarists (but not all and Tony may be an exception here) have particular problems with combining non-health outcomes (such as the impact on patients of reduced waiting times – over and above any health gain from being treated earlier – an improved hospital environment, travel times, and the quality of hospital food) with health outcomes. This is because money valuations of these other elements are needed, which are usually obtained by the use of willingness-to-pay techniques. (Of course this doesn't have to be the case – discrete choice experiments (DCEs) in which people traded health against waiting or the quality of hospital 'hotel services' could in theory be undertaken.) The response of many (but not all) extra-welfarists is often to argue (or simply assume) either that health gain is the only objective of the healthcare system, or that other outcomes (often characterised as 'process' outcomes) are in practice *de minimus* and so can be ignored in any analysis. Others point

(correctly) to some of the practical problems with the use of DCE and contingent valuation techniques – e.g. Dolan and Tsuchiya, Chapter 12

- prefer to see people making choices between social outcomes rather than individual outcomes, and want distributional weights to be applied to QALYs. But where do they come from? Alan's research aimed to generate them from individual preferences, but over different distributional weights, i.e. according to the public policy question. So we need to distinguish revealed/stated preferences for 'private' goods and for publicly provided goods where extra-welfarists can ask public choice questions
- have an interest in 'deliberative processes', which I take to be *forming* preferences through dialogue. It is a political process. On this view we cannot see the political process as one where people simply express preferences through a ballot box. Voting is a preference-revelation exercise only, political debate is a preference-*forming* exercise.

IS EXTRA-WELFARISM AS PRAGMATIC AND ECLECTIC AS IMPLIED AND INDEED WELFARISM AS INCOMPLETE?

Theoretical demands of the *decision-making approach* are in principle strong:

- CEA *can* be compatible with the Paretian approach, i.e. we *could* be doing welfare economics. But strict criteria have to be met (Garber and Phelps, 1997)
- the decision-maker approach needs good valuations of health. Expected utility theory also requires strong conditions to be met – for a discussion see McGuire (2001).

Tony's extra-welfarism is not a route to theoretical laxity. In practice, however, QALYs come from different routes which produce different values (*see* Chapter 10). Parkin and Devlin (2006) comment on the inconsistency between disapproval of the use of VAS (Visual Analogue Scale) and tolerance in comparing studies that use different approaches to QALY determination. Pragmatism is required – which Tony would, I think, support. Welfarists are in danger of being parodied here. They can be eclectic too.

> The most precise definition of a social state would be a complete description of the amount of each type of commodity in the hands of each individual . . . the amount of each productive resource invested in each type of productive activity, *and the amounts of various types of collective activity, such as municipal services, diplomacy and its continuation by other means, and the erection of statues to famous men.*
>
> Arrow (1963, p. 17) (my emphasis)

In other words, seeking individual preferences over bundles of socially provided goods is welfarist.

DOES WELFARISM HAVE NOTHING TO OFFER ON DISTRIBUTIONAL MATTERS?

In principle, welfarist approaches can identify gainers and losers and then (as above) seek individual preferences over different distributions of these gains and losses, i.e. between groups of patients, in the same way as Tony supposes an extra-welfarist would. Of course, there are two concerns for an extra-welfarist:

- any use of willingness to pay to identify gains and losses introduces income constraints into valuations
- there is no use of deliberative processes, i.e. no preference formation only preference elicitation.

More fundamentally, a social welfare function has to be imposed. Extra-welfarists are very comfortable with this and have put much effort into tools to inform and develop society's ability to understand social preferences.

IS THERE A ROLE FOR WELFARISM IN HEALTHCARE RESOURCE ALLOCATION?

Well, as Tony says, 'what is the question, THAT is the answer'. There are perhaps three potential areas where a welfarist approach may answer the question:

- firstly, to support the 'New Labour' efforts to introduce a service orientation (in terms of consumer responsiveness) to public services. Here the question involves understanding public preferences over non-health aspects of NHS service, and measuring the value of healthcare output using monetary valuations of non-health outcomes in combination with a monetary value of health outcomes (which can come from an extra welfarist cost per QALY threshold)
- secondly, with the use of DCE techniques to derive QALYs. Here we are using techniques more normally associated with welfare economics to derive the extra-welfarist measure of health valuation
- thirdly, to address the question of how much should the NHS budget be? (Tony explicitly confines his remarks to resource allocation *within* health care.) Now we need to understand how people trade off health care versus (say) education expenditure or lower taxes. We may be able to use the 'super-QALY' (*see* Chapter 13) to compare the outputs of public services, but some sense of private welfare from the consumption of marketed goods and services is needed to look at the trade-off with taxation.

CONCLUSION

There is a sense in which extra-welfarism is portrayed as a purer approach (in the sense both of more representative of what matters to humans, and in the sense of being fairer as it abstracts from measures constrained by income) but also a pragmatic and eclectic approach, and therefore better designed to give the decision maker the best possible chance of understanding the impact of different policy choices. The reality seems to be a little more complicated. Health care, and some other services, are different. A narrow application of welfarism cannot help with distributional questions. An extra-welfarist approach has clear advantages as a framework for resource allocation in these services. Extra-welfarists also have high methodological standards (although perhaps greater willingness to ignore them – which may or may not be a good thing); many have ambiguous attitudes to preference elicitation; and – in their understandable fear of introducing income constraints through the 'back door' – an aversion to willingness-to-pay techniques that risks inhibiting their ability to support decision makers with pragmatic analysis.

In healthcare resource allocation, extra-welfarism should rule, but welfarist techniques can and should be used to assist in understanding preferences and valuations within an extra-welfarist framework. As Tony implies, the appropriate combination of analytical tools to use depends on 'what is the question'.

REFERENCES

Arrow K (1963) *Social Choice and Individual Values* (2e). New York: John Wiley and Sons.

Arrow K, Solow R, Portney PR *et al.* (1993) Report of the NOAA Panel on Contingent Valuation. *Federal Register* **58**: 4601–14.

Garber A and Phelps C (1997) Economic foundations of cost-effectiveness analysis. *Journal of Health Economics* **16**: 1–31.

McGuire A (2001) Theoretical concepts in the economic evaluation of health care. In: Drummond M and McGuire A (eds) *Economic Evaluation in Health Care*. Oxford: Oxford University Press, pp. 1–21.

Muellbauer J (1987) Professor Sen on the Standard of Living. In: Hawthorn G (ed.) *The Standard of Living*. Cambridge: Cambridge University Press, pp. 39–58.

Parkin D and Devlin N (2006) Is there a case for using visual analogue scale valuations in cost utility analysis? *Health Economics* **15**: 653–64.

Sen A (1987a) The standard of living: Lecture I, Concepts and critiques. In: Hawthorn G (ed.) *The Standard of Living*. Cambridge: Cambridge University Press, pp. 1–19.

Sen A (1987b) The standard of living: Lecture II, Lives and capabilities. In: Hawthorn G (ed.) *The Standard of Living*. Cambridge: Cambridge University Press, pp. 20–38.

Sen A (2002) Health: perception versus observation. *British Medical Journal* **324**: 860–1.

ACKNOWLEDGEMENTS

I would like to thank Diane Dawson, Anne Mason, Nancy Devlin and Tony Culyer for very helpful comments.

CHAPTER 8

Being reasonable about equity and fairness: looking back and extending the Williams way

... Aki Tsuchiya and Paul Dolan

This paper begins with a brief introduction looking at the general background on equity and fairness in health and health care (independently of Alan Williams' work), and then moves on to an overview of Alan's work in the area. Then the main part of the paper will cover three topics, all centring on the fair innings argument. First, the fair innings argument in general will be explained, using static social class weights and dynamic age weights as an example. Second, the formal process of deriving each of these weights using a health-related social welfare function is presented. Third, its application to the inequality in health between the sexes, and the possibility of going beyond health will be examined. Building on the work left by Alan, the paper will conclude with what we think are the next topics of research in this area.

INTRODUCTION: EQUITY AND FAIRNESS IN HEALTH AND HEALTH CARE

Equity and fairness in standard textbooks

Let us begin by carrying out a brief and informal review of how the topic of equity and fairness in health and health care has been treated in standard textbooks or introductory texts of health economics (or, at least, in the textbooks that we have used in our own teaching). The reason for starting with textbooks is because it seems to be a quick and reasonable way to identify the core issues and questions in the discipline: health economists may not agree on *how* to answer these but there may be some broad agreement on *what* are the issues that need addressing.

The Economics of Health Care: an introductory text, by Alistair McGuire, John Henderson and Gavin Mooney was published in 1988. It consists of 12 chapters, one of which is about 'Distribution'. The importance of consideration for equity in health care is already introduced in an earlier chapter on 'Health care as an economic commodity', and this chapter discusses the reasons why equity is important. Equity is defined as 'involving some conscious departures(s) from the pursuit of maximising welfare (subject to some budget constraint) in the interest of a more equal distribution of some health-related characteristic (e.g. health care utilisation)' (McGuire *et al*, 1988, p.55; brackets in original).* Two concepts of equity are introduced: equity as equal access for equal need (which is presented as the key policy concern), and equity as equal mortality and morbidity across socio-economically defined population groups (which is what measurement is usually concerned about). The main part of the chapter is devoted to reviewing various reasons why equity matters, including altruism, sympathy, the Kantian moral imperative, Sen's commitment, and Rawlsian maximin, and how they apply to health care in the real world. While there is explicit acknowledgement that equity may conflict with efficiency, the focus of the chapter is on the relationships between the different theories of equity.

The second edition of *Economics, Medicine and Health Care* by Gavin Mooney was published in 1992 (first edition 1986). The book has two chapters out of ten where the central theme is on equity and fairness in health care. (In addition, the issue of fair shares is discussed in another chapter on financing.) The first of the two chapters questions the relevance of medical ethics in health care. Interestingly, the so-called conflict between medical ethics and economics is reformulated as a conflict between norms at the individual decision level and norms at the societal decision level. The following chapter explicitly addresses the issue of equity and fairness in health care (at the societal, or economic, level). The question of 'what is equity', or how to operationalise equity in health care, is addressed and seven rival definitions are compared ranging from equity as the equal expenditure per capita, equity as equal access for equal need, to equity as equality of health across individuals; and how they conflict with each other. The objective is not to promote a particular definition, but to highlight the confusion that arises from uncritical use of different definitions of equity. There is also explicit recognition that the pursuit of equity may conflict with efficiency goals.

Distributing Health Care: economic and ethical issues by Paul Dolan and Jan Abel Olsen was published in 2002. As the title suggests, distributional and ethical issues are central to the book, with three chapters out of nine specifically dedicated towards them. There is an extensive discussion on the 'equity of what', or what the distribuendum is: utility, primary goods, capabilities, or health. For the main part of the book, equity is operationalised as the equality of health, and competing approaches such as sum ranking, maximin, and egalitarianism are interpreted as providing support for different points along the utility possibility frontier; in other words, the pursuit of equity need not

* This definition is problematic. It rules out cases where an unequal distribution might be more equitable. However, the text further down the same page recognises that vertical equity involves the unequal treatment of unequals.

involve a trade-off with Pareto efficiency.* This culminates in the application of equity weights to quality-adjusted life years (QALYs) in cost-effectiveness analyses. Neither equity as equality of access nor equity as equality of utilisation is discussed in this book. Alongside the heavily consequentialist flavour of equity as equality of health, there is an extensive discussion of procedural justice, 'which posits that the fairness of the procedures used in a decision-making process will influence an individual's reaction to the decision' (Dolan and Olsen, 2002, p. 44).

The fourth edition of *The Economics of Health and Health Care* by Sherman Folland, Allen Goodman and Miron Stano was published in 2004. There is one chapter out of 24 on 'Equity, efficiency, and need'. It devotes little space to the debate on 'what is equity', and the term 'equity' does not appear in the glossary. The main part of the chapter assumes the answer to the question of 'equity of what' is utility, as opposed to health or health care, but later parts explore alternative theories including equal opportunities and maximin.

The last textbook reviewed here is the second edition of *Economics of Health Care Financing: the visible hand* by Cam Donaldson and Karen Gerard, which was published in 2005. There are two chapters addressing equity and fairness. The first of these, on economic objectives of health care, reinterprets the ongoing debate on 'what is equity' as one concerning horizontal equity, and point out that there is another, vertical version of equity, namely the equity of financial contribution to health care: in essence, the rich should contribute more towards the finance of health care than the poor.† The authors state their own view 'that equity objectives should be focused on health care [such as equity regarding access, utilisation, and/or finance] rather than health' (Donaldson and Gerard, 2005, p. 87; square brackets added). There is also a brief mention of procedural justice. The second chapter on equity reviews evidence on the distribution of contribution to healthcare finance and of opportunities to utilise health care.

From this brief review‡ we will conclude that there are three core questions in equity and fairness in health and health care (also see Wagstaff and van Doorslaer, 2000).

First core question: what is equity of health care?

Equity in health care can be defined either as the equality of expenditure,

* However, Dolan and Olsen (2002) continue to discuss trade-offs between efficiency and equity in the context of health-related social welfare functions. The implication is that the definition of efficiency in use is not Paretian but utilitarian.

† This formulation is problematic. For example, *ceteris paribus*, horizontal equity requires that those with equal income make equal contributions to the finance of health care, and vertical equity requires that those with unequal need receive unequal health care.

‡ There is also a forthcoming textbook by Stephen Morris, Nancy Devlin and David Parkin. Judging by the list of contents on a promotion flyer by Wiley, there will be one chapter out of eleven devoted to 'equity in health care'.

access, utilisation, or health benefit, controlling for need;* or, alternatively, equity in health care can be equality of health. This debate goes back to Mooney (1983), and was revisited by Culyer and Wagstaff (1993). The health economists' community seems to be split roughly into those who argue for equity as equality of access (who may use utilisation as a proxy for access) and those who argue for equity as equality of health. The latter include those who appreciate equal access as an immediate objective as long as it contributes towards achieving equal health. Each school is related to a large empirical literature overlapping with public health, reporting the evidence on the extent to which equity is or is not achieved.

Second core question: equity of what?

Those who support the idea of health as the distribuendum face a two-pronged attack. Besides the debate above against those who believe in the equity of healthcare services as opposed to the equity of health, they also face those who assume that the distribuendum is utility, not health. This question as to what to equalise across the relevant population relates to ideology. The welfarist tradition has held that the distribuendum addressed in economics is individual utility. Non-welfarism in health economics began by putting forward health as the distribuendum, but this may be because health was counted as one of the basic capabilities that people should have opportunities to achieve (Culyer, 1989; also see Cookson, 2005). On the other hand, challenging consequentialist foundations of standard welfare economics has led to questioning *distributive* justice as the only criterion for equity, and to arguing for *procedural* justice in health care (Tsuchiya *et al.*, 2005).

Third core question: what is financial equity?

Financial equity is defined as unequal contribution to healthcare finance, in proportion to income. It seems to be a much less controversial topic,† and a large part of the literature concerns methods on how to operationalise this concept, and evidence on the extent to which different countries and healthcare systems achieve financial equity.

Overview of Alan Williams' contribution to the literature

Let us look at Alan's views on the three core questions identified above. Alan's position was that what matters is the equity of health, or equality in lifetime experiences of health across different population groups. Equity in terms of health care (access or finance) is an instrumental means that contribute

* And of course, there is the debate on what is need. The two rival definitions are: the capacity to benefit, and ill-health *per se*.

† It also seems possible to define financial equity as contribution to healthcare finance in proportion to the volume of heathcare services consumed, or in proportion to the size of health benefit achieved, but neither seem to be debated. This is probably because the former is in effect the free market, i.e. the default model in microeconomics, and the latter may be interesting but in reality totally impractical.

towards achieving the more fundamental equity objective, equality of life time health. After all, the *efficiency* objective of any healthcare system is to maximise health, not to maximise healthcare delivery *per se*. Health care is of value to the extent that it improves health. If so, why should the *equity* objective be about health care as opposed to health? A good example is the *Handbook of Health Economics* chapter with Richard Cookson on 'Equity in health' (Williams and Cookson, 2000). All the figures representing different approaches to equity are about health between two parties, because health is the distribuendum.

Alan's work on equity in health can be divided roughly into three groups. The first group of work is *theoretical*, which overlaps with political and moral philosophy. Besides his *Handbook of Health Economics* chapter this group includes a paper subtitled 'A guide though the ideological jungle', where libertarian and egalitarian views are contrasted, and discussed in the context of public and private funding of health care (Williams, 1988a). Then, there is an interesting exchange with the utilitarian philosopher John Harris who criticised 'QALYfying' peoples' life, and the use of simple aggregation rules across different patients in healthcare resource allocation (Harris, 1987). Alan's reply was succinct and summarised the differences between Harris's position and his own (Williams, 1987). In a paper presented to the Royal Institute of Philosophy Conference on 'Philosophy and Medical Welfare' in 1987, and published as a monograph in the following year, Alan questions whether or not the societal value of a unit of health should be regarded as equal across all types of patient, and proposes several possibilities to be explored in survey work. This list includes discrimination (or differential weighting) by age, by family responsibilities, by social worth (or talent), by individual choice and behaviour, by deprivation, and (just to see whether people support it) by willingness and ability to pay (Williams, 1988). Leading on from this, the most important piece of theoretical work by Alan in this area is probably the one on the fair innings argument (Williams, 1997); this will be discussed in more detail below.

The second group of work overlaps with public health, and is about finding out the *facts* (the extent and determinants) of existing inequalities in lifetime health across different population groups within different countries. A large part of this enterprise was carried out in collaboration with members of the EuroQol Group. The MVH (Measurement and Valuation of Health) study reported population norms for the UK using the EQ-5D instrument (Kind *et al.*, 1998). More recently, Szende and Williams (2004) looked at the differences in self-reported health using the EQ-5D instrument across 15 different countries; they disaggregated this by age, gender and educational attainment; and reported inequalities in health at the individual level and disaggregated by the dimensions of EQ-5D.

The third group of work involves eliciting *values*: i.e. finding out what people think about the existing inequality in lifetime health across population groups, and to what extent people will trade off efficiency in order to improve equity.

This belongs to an area of work that some call 'empirical ethics'. Alan often used participants of public health or health policy conferences he attended, and audiences of health economics lectures he gave, as guinea pigs (see for example the relevant sections in Williams, 1988b; or Williams *et al.*, 2005). In a research area where large-scale surveys of representative samples of the general public are often seen as the only sound way ahead, Alan was impatient because imperfect data now has its uses and perfect data may never materialise. In a more formal project funded by the Economic and Social Research Council (ESRC) on 'Measuring preferences regarding equity and variations in health', Alan (and both of the authors of this paper) contributed towards quantifying the trade-off that members of the public will make between improving overall average health and reducing inequalities between different population groups (Shaw *et al.*, 2001; Dolan *et al.*, 2002; Dolan and Tsuchiya, 2003; Williams *et al.*, 2005). The findings from this project will be revisited below.

THE FAIR INNINGS ARGUMENT IN HEALTH ECONOMICS

History of the concept and the *Health Economics* 1997 paper

In 1987, Alan had a debate in the *Journal of Medical Ethics* with John Harris. It therefore came as a surprise to some of us who were aware of this bit of history that at the first International Health Economics Association conference at Vancouver in 1996 Alan gave a plenary talk, which was based on John Harris' idea in his 1985 book *The Value of Life*. This was the fair innings argument, and the talk was subsequently published in *Health Economics* (Williams, 1997). The quote from *The Value of Life* which Alan used summarises the essence of the fair innings argument: 'while it is always a *misfortune* to die when one wants to go on living, it is not a *tragedy* to die in old age; but it is on the other hand both a tragedy and a misfortune to be cut off prematurely' (Harris, 1985, p. 93; cited in Williams, 1997; italics in original). However, Alan has been thinking about discriminating against elderly people in a transparent and systematic manner at least as far back as 1987 (Williams, 1988b).

Similar ethical views have been discussed in the bioethics literature by Jonathan Glover (1977), Norman Daniels (1988), Michael Lockwood (1988), and Daniel Callahan (1990; see Tsuchiya, 2000a, for a review). The innovation by Alan introduced a clear trade-off with efficiency, so that the intensity of this argument can be expressed in terms of the magnitude of overall health gain that can be sacrificed for it, which was in stark contrast to the approaches taken by the philosophers.

In the 1997 paper in *Health Economics*, Alan argues that everybody should be entitled to some common target quantity of lifetime health, ideally measured in terms of QALYs. If some die without having achieved this fair innings, then they are in some sense 'cheated'. Then, he introduces an inequality-averse health-related social welfare function, deriving a rate of substitution between a marginal health improvement to one group (whose lifetime health is expected to exceed the fair innings) and a marginal health improvement to another group (whose lifetime health is expected to fall short of the fair innings); this value can then be used as the basis of an equity weight in healthcare priority setting.

The paper used the example of UK men from different socio-economic classes. The first stage was *static*, and based on quality-adjusted life expectancy at birth (QALE(0); this is based on the usual life table adjusted for the level of health at different ages): men from social classes I and II have a QALE(0) of 66 years, whereas men from social classes IV and V have a QALE(0) of 57 years. Therefore, other things being the same, a marginal health gain to the former will be valued less by society than a marginal health gain to the latter. So at this point, the fair innings argument is being used to generate social class weights.

The next stage was to make this *dynamic*. At any point in time, within any given population subgroup, expected age of death is an increasing function of age due to the survivor effect. Thus, if 20 year olds and 60 year olds from the same socio-economic background are compared, the 60 year olds will have a higher expected age of death (and therefore expected lifetime QALYs, or ELQ). Applying the fair innings argument to this situation will lead to the conclusion that, other things being the same, the social value of a marginal health improvement to 20 year olds is larger than the same to a 60 year old. This then is the fair innings age weighting (within a given socio-economic class).

The third stage was to look at the effect of across-class *and* across-age fair innings weights. Since those in social classes I and II at birth are already expected to achieve the (provisional) fair innings of 61 QALYs, whereas those in social classes IV and V are not expected to achieve this until they reach age 64 years, the impact of social class is found to be larger than the impact of age.* In other words, if the comparison is between young people from social classes I and II and old people from social classes IV and V, the effect of class will be much stronger, so that the older group will get a larger fair innings weight unless they are over 80 years and have achieved an ELQ of above 67 QALYs (*see* Table 4 of Williams, 1997). Also note that all Alan's examples are for marginal health benefits where the current population lifetime health prospects apply to the patients in question. Instead, in the case of young people from social classes I and II and old people from social classes IV and V *who are all about to die without treatment*, then since the former group has much smaller ELQ without treatment compared to the latter group, their weights will be larger to reflect this. This time, it is the age factor that determines the weights rather than the class factor.

---

* In this respect, it is interesting why Alan should have promoted the fair innings weights as a tool for intergenerational equity rather than interclass equity.

Fair innings weights and the health-related social welfare function*

The general setting

While the above ideas were explored in the *Health Economics* 1997 paper, the latter did not include an explicit exposition on how exactly the static and dynamic weights are to be derived, or how they are related to each other. This section is an attempt to fill that gap.

Suppose there is an extra QALY that could be given to one of two patient groups of the same size at equal cost, and that the only difference between these two groups is their lifetime health prospect without treatment, such that those in one group have 70 ELQ(0) while those in the other group have 50 ELQ. The two axes of Figure 8.1 represent ELQ(0) of the two groups. It shows the current situation at point *P*, where ELQ(0) of the two population subgroups *a* and *b* are H_{a0} and H_{b0} respectively. Point *A* represents the average of the two ELQs, or 'overall health'. Point *P′* is the situation where H_{a0} and H_{b0} are interchanged. Assuming symmetry, the level of social welfare at points *P* and *P′* are identical. Now, suppose that members of the general public are presented with a description of the present situation *P* and asked how much overall health, in terms of QALYs, they would be willing to forego (WTF) for an equal distribution between the two population subgroups. This will lead to the determination of the level of the fair innings: i.e. average health minus the WTF.† Point *E* on the 45° line is where both populations have an ELQ(0) equal to the level of fair innings. The implication is that people are indifferent between the three points *P*, *P′*, and *E*, and thus these points must lie on the same social welfare contour. Figure 8.2 illustrates such a curve.

While there can be more than one specification that yields an iso-welfare curve through these three points, let us assume a health-related social welfare function (HRSWF) that is increasing in subgroup health and has constant elasticity of substitution so that:

$$W = \left[\alpha H_{ax}^{-r} + (1-\alpha)\mathrm{H}_{bx}^{-r}\right]^{-\frac{1}{r}},\ H_a, H_b > 0, r \neq 0 \text{ [eq. 1]},$$

where *W* represents the level of health-related social welfare, and *r* represents the curvature of the HRSWF so that when there is aversion to inequality, then $r > -1$ and the iso-welfare curve becomes convex to the origin. This value can be obtained from observed values for FI, H_{ax}, and H_{bx}. When WTF = 0, then r = –1. This is the case of the classical utilitarian HRSWF, which implies neutrality over distribution, and individual QALY gains are summed together with no weights attached.

The α and $1-\alpha$ parameters indicate the rates at which the health of the two

---

* This section draws on a Health Economists' Study Group (HESG) paper presented at Newcastle some time ago (Tsuchiya, 2000b).

† In other words, the fair innings is the equally distributed equivalent *health*.

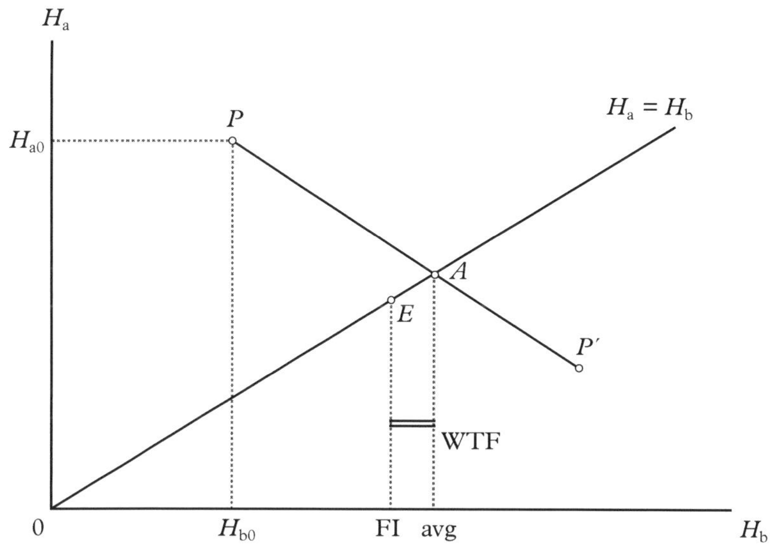

FIGURE 8.1 The present situation and WTF. avg, average expected lifetime QALYs = overall health; FI, the fair innings; WTF, willingness to forego overall health for more equal distribution; *A*, the point at which both parties achieve average health; *E*, the point at which both parties achieve the fair innings.

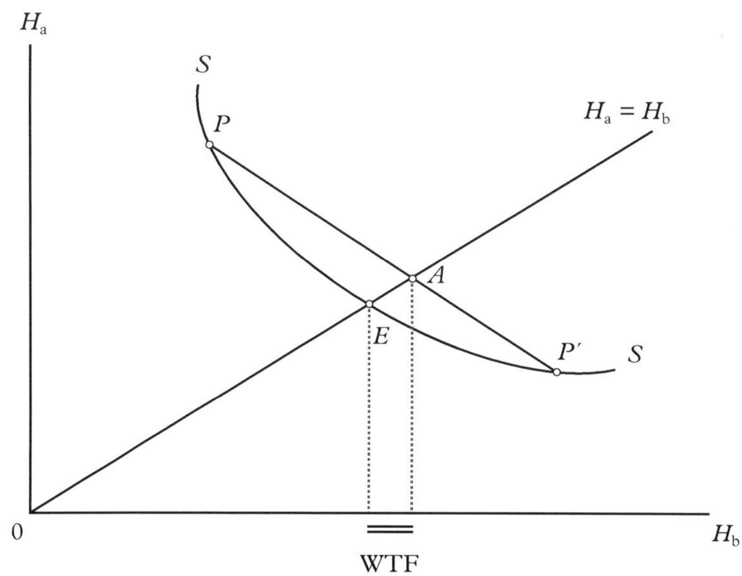

FIGURE 8.2 The social welfare contour. *A*, the point at which both parties achieve average health; *E*, the point at which both parties achieve the fair innings; *SS*, the social welfare contour.

population subgroups enter the social welfare calculus. So, if the health of the two population subgroups were perceived to be of different social worth (e.g. because one group is responsible for their own poor health), then $\alpha \neq 1 - \alpha$ to reflect this. Where the assumption is that neither party is responsible for the difference in lifetime health, $\alpha = 1 - \alpha = ½$. While on the one hand r influences the rate at which the health of a population subgroup affects social welfare based on how healthy that group is compared to the other, regardless of all other attributes of these groups, α on the other hand influences the rate at which the health of the subgroups affects social welfare depending on who these people are, regardless of their levels of health relative to each other.*

The static model: relative subgroup weights at birth

The static weight for subgroup *a* relative to *b* at a given point $P(H_{a0},H_{b0})$ is to reflect, under constant social welfare, the relative value of a marginal increase in the health of subgroup *a* in terms of a marginal increase in the health of subgroup *b*, which in Figure 8.3 corresponds to the negative inverse of the tangent *TT* at point *P*. This is the inverse of the marginal rate of substitution (MRS) between H_a and H_b, and thus static weight $SW_{a:b}$ can be represented as:

$$SW_{a:b} \equiv -\frac{dH_{b0}}{dH_{a0}} \quad \text{[eq. 2a].}$$

Since, by definition, $dW = 0$ along the iso-welfare contour,

$$-\frac{dH_{b0}}{dH_{a0}} = \frac{\partial W/\partial H_{a0}}{\partial W/\partial H_{b0}}$$

and substituting this into [eq. 2a] yields the static weight:

$$SW_{a:b} = \frac{\alpha}{1-\alpha}\left[\frac{H_{b0}}{H_{a0}}\right]^{(1+r)},$$

where, under assumption $\alpha = 1 - \alpha$:

$$SW_{a:b} = [H_{b0}/H_{a0}]^{(1+r)} \quad \text{[eq. 2b].}$$

* There may be several factors that affect the value of α and whether or not $\alpha = 1 - \alpha$. One candidate is the effect of individual choice and liability, so that for example one group will be smokers and the other group will be non-smokers. If, by appropriate means, it can be established that different people are responsible by varying degrees for some aspects of their own lifetime health, and if this magnitude is quantified, then the α parameter can be estimated and incorporated in the model.

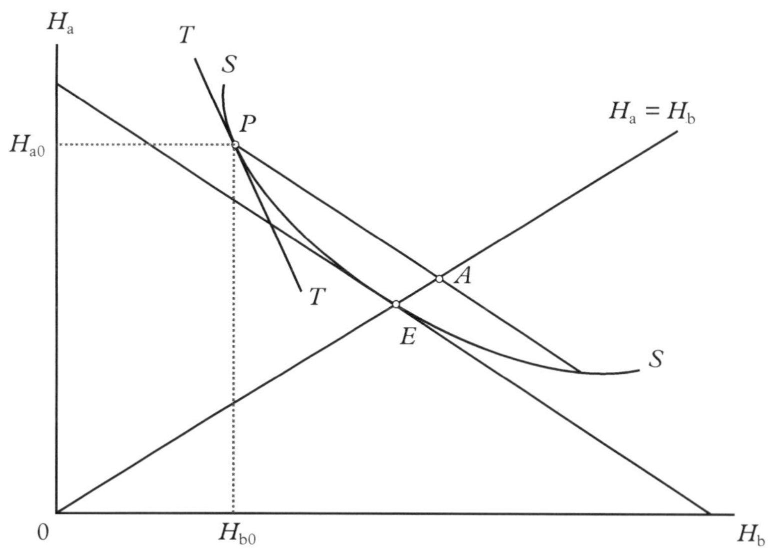

FIGURE 8.3 Static weights for subgroups *a* and *b*. *A*, the point at which both parties achieve average health; *E*, the point at which both parties achieve the fair innings; *SS*, the social welfare contour; line *TT* is the tangent to the contour at point *P*.

Note that the subscript of *SW* includes the reference subgroup, reflecting the fact that this weight is relative to the health of the comparator subgroup, in this case *b*, and therefore, not independent of how other subgroups fare in terms of ELQ. Further, it does not specify age. These subgroup weights thus obtained are static in the sense that they are calculated based on ELQ(0) regardless of present age, past QALYs, present QALE, or present ELQ of those involved, and thus everybody in the same subgroup is given the same weight. Static weights have been defined in the 1997 paper and calculated with reference to ELQ at birth, but these may also be calculated for ELQ at any given age.

The dynamic model: subgroup-and-age-specific weights

The dynamic weight specific to population subgroup n at age x can reflect the increase in ELQ with age by basing the calculation on H_{nx} instead of H_{n0}. Unless one acquires a disability that is significant both in terms of severity and duration, most people's ELQ improves with age (or with survival). Dynamic weights take into account the effect of increasing ELQ through survival, so that the larger one's ELQ, the smaller will be the weight given to one's marginal health improvement. Incorporation of such weights into cost–QALY analyses will imply that, other things being equal, the older one is, the healthcare treatment one receives has to clear an increasingly lower cost per QALY threshold than that for a younger candidate patient. Although the fair innings weights can be interpreted as age weights under an 'other-things-being-equal' clause, strictly speaking, they are not *age* weights but weights by ELQ.*

The actual weight is calculated with reference to the standard prospect of achieving a given fair innings, which makes this weight relatively independent of ELQ of other subgroups so long as the level of the fair innings itself remains the same. The dynamic weight (*DW*) is calculated by substituting FI_r (the level of fair innings given *r*) for H_b and H_{nx} for H_a of [eq. 2b]:

$$DW_{nx} = [FI_r/H_{nx}]^{(1+r)} \quad \text{[eq. 3]}.$$

This is the most general formula that allows to deal with cases where $n > 2$ without any adjustments. Further, the relative subgroup static weight $SW_{n:m}$ at birth can be obtained by dividing DW_{n0} by DW_{m0}.

Figure 8.4 depicts three cases where the fixed prospect of achieving the fair innings is represented on the horizontal axes (subgroup *b*), and ELQ at age *x* of subgroup *a* is (1) smaller than, (2) equal to, and (3) larger than the fair innings. The figure shows two things: that DW_{nx} is larger (smaller) than 1 when ELQ is smaller (larger) than the fair innings; and that the calculation of DW_{nx} corresponding to different ELQs involves more than one contour of the same SWF.

The 1997 paper justifies this involvement of different levels of *W* to obtain dynamic weights by an argument which in effect states that: since it is unlikely that we will actually find ourselves on the production possibility frontier, the frontier can be ignored. It can also be argued that since it is the MRS between two potential health improvements, and since MRS belongs to the realm of preferences and not resources or production technologies, the production possibility frontier is irrelevant even when it is known for certain that the point lies outside the frontier. The strength of these arguments at the practical level may depend on how feasible it is to picture being at point (H_{ax}, FI_r). Where the difference in health between the subgroups is very large and the subgroup in question is the healthier one, this point may become increasingly implausible, not on theoretical grounds, but on practical grounds (because H_{bx} is so much lower than FI_r).

One may further want to question the legitimacy of comparing, for example, DW_{a20} with DW_{b60}: i.e. the dynamic weight given to 20 year olds in subgroup *a*, and the dynamic weight given to 60 year olds in subgroup *b*. These two weights will be derived from the same SWF, but from two different contours of this: i.e. DW_{a20} is based on the gradient of the contour at (H_{a20}, FI_r) and DW_{b60} comes from the gradient of another contour at (FI_r, H_{b60}). Does it make sense to compare gradients from two different contours, and therefore

* For instance, an individual that acquires a significant permanent disability at middle age will record a sharp drop in ELQ at that point, and therefore his/her weight will sharply increase accordingly. Further, if the disability stays stable, his/her weights will gradually decrease from then onwards, with age, but at a slower rate than the weights of those without permanent disabilities.

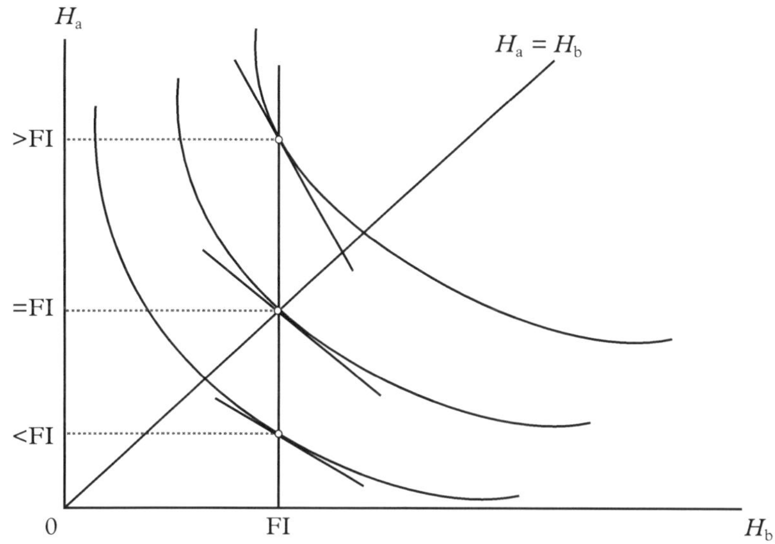

FIGURE 8.4 Dynamic weights for subgroup *a*.

relate to different levels of social welfare? However, on a theoretical level, it is always possible to identify a point (H_a, H_b), where $H_a = H_{a20}$ and $H_b = H_{b60}$, and, since static weights do not refer to age *x per se*, $SW_{a:b}$ at this point will coincide with the ratio between DW_{a20} and DW_{b60}. In other words, the gradient of the contour through this point will correspond to comparing DW_{a20} and DW_{b60}, and therefore, the direct comparison of these two can legitimately be made. At an empirical level, the concern translates to the issue of whether or not the value of *r* is constant for all possible combinations of (H_a, H_b). In other words, whether or not the preferences elicited from the general public will be as well behaved as expected by theory. This is an important issue that goes beyond the scope of this paper.

Fair innings and the sex problem: from health to wider well-being

When faced with the question why equity of health and not equity of health care, Alan seems to have had two thoughts. The first is mentioned above: because improving health is the final objective of healthcare services. The equity objective is equality of health, where equity of health care might be a means towards achieving this end. The second is because health measured in ELQ is the variable that seems to best reflect the people's well-being. Those who are richer, better educated, better nourished, with more socio-economic opportunities, more privileged, and happier all live longer and healthier lives than those who are not . . . but there is a caveat to this: provided the comparison is within the same sex group. Women in most societies live longer (and have larger ELQ) than men, although they are poorer, less educated, have fewer socio-economic opportunities and are less privileged than men.* So, when comparing across the gender groups, health no longer seems to work as the one variable to represent people's well-being.

In the ESRC project on 'Measuring preferences regarding equity and variations in health', we explained to members of the public that there is a five-year difference in life expectancy at birth between men from social classes I and V. When respondents were asked in effect for the size of the WTF in order to reduce this gap in life expectancy, the median answer was 1 year. When the same respondents were told that there is the same five-year gap in life expectancy at birth between men and women, however, the median WTF was zero (Dolan *et al.*, 2002). If the fair innings argument is valid, then shouldn't the respondents want to make some sacrifices in efficiency in order to rectify this gap in life expectancy? Or, could it be that the fair innings argument will work across social classes (and across different ages), but not across the gender groups?

In a theoretical paper, Tsuchiya and Williams (2004) explored reasons why people's attitude towards inequality in health might differ between the social class scenario and the gender scenario, and whether this seriously limits the applicability of the fair innings argument. The main conclusion is that if people are taking into account some notion of overall well-being that stretches beyond health and longevity, then they may think that although men have lower ELQ, they may not necessarily have a lower level of overall well-being, because of the other socio-economic advantages they have over women. If so, then men are not the relatively worse off amongst the two sexes, so it will not be equitable to give a marginal health improvement to men a higher relative weight than the same health improvement to women. This has two implications. First, it may be inappropriate to apply the fair innings argument to *health* across the sex groups, but that does not mean the fair innings argument cannot be applied to *overall well-being* across the sex groups. Second, WTF and the fair innings weights derived in the above study between the social classes may be overestimated, since those in social class V have fewer socio-economic opportunities than those in social class I, and this consideration (over and above the consideration for their poorer health) may have had a positive impact on WTF.

FUTURE RESEARCH PRIORITIES

We see three main directions for research following from all of this. One direction is descriptive and involves collaboration with public health researchers. Investigation into the determinants of ELQ, and the determinants of the

* Women live longer than men even in societies where they are less well nourished. Would a genderless society, where sexism was overcome, be one where women lived yet longer than men? Probably not, since it seems to be that patriarchal societies are bad for men's health and longevity as well as women's (*see* for example Kawachi *et al.*, 1999; Stanistreet *et al.*, 2005).

variation of ELQ, are two important topics. Related to these is the measurement of inequality across different population subgroups.

Another direction involves economic theory and empirical work: the ESRC-funded project mentioned above elicited WTF *independently* for social class, age groups, gender and individual responsibility. Thus, public preferences support giving larger weights to those from deprived backgrounds, and those who are young, and those who have not caused their own ill-health. But what should we do about somebody who is from a deprived background *and* old *and* may have caused their own ill-health? We need to look at combinations of relevant characteristics, not just one characteristic at a time. There is a research programme, where we have one of the two major research projects, currently funded by NICE and the National Collaboration Centre for Research Methodology on 'The relative societal value of health gains to different beneficiaries' to explore this topic further.

The third is about expanding beyond health economics, into the economics of well-being, to explore the extent to which non-welfarism can be applied in other areas of public policy beyond health and health care. One such attempt has been discussed in our other paper at this conference on public safety. The aim there is to generate a descriptive system to capture the impact of crime on individual well-being, and to produce a population value set that goes with it. Similar attempts may be made in other areas of public policy where non-welfarist approaches may enjoy support such as social care, education, environment, and defence. This expansion will not stop at measuring and valuing well-being, but will also include the application of the fair innings weights and the derivation of distributional weights applicable to the different components of well-being, or indeed to well-being overall.

REFERENCES

Callahan D (1990) *What kind of life: the limits of medical progress*. Georgetown: University Press.

Cookson R (2005) QALYs and the capabilities approach. *Health Economics* **14**: 817–29.

Culyer AJ (1989) The normative economics of health care finance and provision. *Oxford Review of Economic Policy* **5**: 34–58.

Culyer AJ and Wagstaff A (1993) Equity and equality in health and health care. *Journal of Health Economics* **12**: 431–57.

Daniels N (1988) *Am I my Parents' Keeper? An essay on justice between the young and the old.* New York: Oxford University Press.

Dolan P and Olsen JA (2002), *Distributing Health Care: economic and ethical issues.* Oxford: Oxford University Press.

Dolan P, Tsuchiya A, Smith P, Shaw R and Williams A (2002) *Determining the Parameters in a Social Welfare Function using Stated Preference Data: an application to health.* Sheffield Health Economics Group Discussion Paper. Sheffield: University of Sheffield.

Dolan P and Tsuchiya A (2003) *The Social Welfare Function and Individual Responsibility: some theoretical issues and empirical evidence from health*, Sheffield Health Economics Group Discussion Paper. Sheffield: University of Sheffield.

Donaldson C and Gerard K (2005) *Economics of Health Care Financing: the visible hand* (2e with Jan S, Mitton C and Wiseman V). Houndmills: Palgrave Macmillan.

Folland S, Goodman AC and Stano M (2004) *The Economics of Health and Health Care* (4e). Upper Saddle River, NJ: Pearson Prentice Hall.

Glover J (1977) *Causing Death and Saving Lives*. Harmondsworth: Penguin.

Harris J (1985) *The Value of Life: an introduction to medical ethics*. London: Routledge.

Harris J (1987) QALYfying the value of life. *Journal of Medical Ethics* **13**: 117–23.

Kawachi I, Kennedy BP, Gupta V and Prothrow-Stith D (1999) Women's status and the health of women and men: a view from the States. *Social Science and Medicine* **48**: 21–32.

Kind P, Dolan P, Gudex C and Williams A (1998) Variations in population health status: results from a United Kingdom national questionnaire survey. *British Medical Journal* **316**: 736–41.

Lockwood M (1988) Quality of life and resource allocation. In: Bell JM and Mendus S (eds). *Philosophy and Medical Welfare*. New York: Cambridge University Press, pp. 33–56.

McGuire A, Henderson J and Mooney G (1988) *The Economics of Health Care: an introductory text*. New York: Routledge.

Mooney G (1983) Equity in health care: confronting the confusion. *Effective Health Care* **1**: 179–85.

Mooney G (1992) *Economics, Medicine and Health Care* (2e). Hemel Hempstead: Harvester Wheatsheaf.

Shaw R, Dolan P, Tsuchiya A *et al.* (2001) *Development of a Questionnaire to Elicit People's Preferences regarding Health Inequalities*. Occasional Paper, Centre for Health Economics. York: University of York.

Stanistreet D, Bambra C, Scott-Samuel A (2005) Is patriarchy the source of men's higher mortality? *Journal of Epidemiology and Community Health* **59**: 873–6.

Szende A and Williams A (eds) (2004) *Measuring Self-reported Population Health: an international perspective based on EQ-5D*. Budapest: Spring Med Publishing.

Tsuchiya A (2000a) QALYs and ageism: philosophical theories and age weighting. *Health Economics* **9**: 57–68.

Tsuchiya A (2000b) *The Design and Calculation of the Fair Innings Weights*, paper presented at the Health Economists' Study Group meeting, Newcastle upon Tyne, 5–7 January.

Tsuchiya A, Miguel LS, Edlin R, Wailoo A and Dolan P (2005) NICE and procedural justice. *Journal of Applied Health Economics and Policy* **4**: 119–27.

Tsuchiya A and Williams A (2004) A 'fair innings' between the sexes? Are men being treated inequitably? *Social Science and Medicine* **60**: 277–86.

Wagstaff A and van Doorslaer E (2000) Equity in health care finance and delivery. In: Culyer AJ and Newhouse JP (eds) *Handbook of Health Economics* vol. 1B. Amsterdam: Elsevier, pp. 1803–62.

Williams A (1987) Response: QALYfying the value of life. *Journal of Medical Ethics* **13**: 123.

Williams A (1988a) Priority setting in public and private health care: a guide through the ideological jungle. *Journal of Health Economics* 7: 173–83.

Williams A (1988b) Ethics and efficiency in the provision of health care. In: Bell JM and Mendus S (eds) *Philosophy and Medical Welfare.* New York: Cambridge University Press, pp. 111–26.

Williams A (1997) Intergenerational equity: an exploration of the 'fair innings argument'. *Health Economics* **6**: 117–32.

Williams A and Cookson R (2000) Equity in health. In: Culyer AJ and Newhouse JP (eds) *Handbook of Health Economics* vol. 1B. Amsterdam: Elsevier, pp. 1863–910.

Williams A, Dolan P and Tsuchiya A (2005) Eliciting equity-efficiency trade offs in health. In: Smith PC, Ginnelly L and Sculpher M (eds) *Health Policy and Economics: Opportunities and Challenges.* Maidenhead: Open University Press, 64–87.

CHAPTER 9

Equity and fairness in health and health care: looking up and extending 'My way' – a comment on Aki Tsuchiya and Paul Dolan's paper

... Jan Abel Olsen

INTRODUCTION

I greatly enjoyed Aki and Paul's overview of Alan's contribution to this literature and their discussion of the fair innings argument. My discussion concentrates on the three core questions they outline, and my main points are related to the importance of acknowledging the very disparate *causes of inequalities* in health when we talk about equity and fairness in health and health *care*.

First, let me try to make my own conceptual clarifications. As opposed to the term efficiency where economists have precise definitions, different disciplines and schools of thought appear to have various definitions of equity and fairness. I will not suggest which definitions are the most precise, but rather which connotations I get – when looking up in the sky. I consider *equity* to deal with *distributive justice*, often with the aim of reducing observed inequalities among people in their possessions of particular goods (e.g. income, health, education). I consider *fairness* to be a wider term, related to what most people think is intuitively right or *acceptable*,* often with reference to particular ethical norms and/or a wide community consensus ('empirical ethics'), and it may have connotations of *procedural justice*. Note also the seminal paper by Rawls (1958) entitled 'Justice as fairness'. In the context of *distributive justice*, I feel that the term *fairness* differs from the term *equity*, in the sense that fairness

* A paper by Kahneman *et al.* (1986) 'Fairness as a constraint on profit seeking: entitlement in the market', reports from a survey in which the various statements were labelled 'acceptable' versus 'unfair'.

also includes, and refers to, the ethical justifications for accepting particular inequalities.

It appears that Aki and Paul are primarily concerned with equity rather than fairness. The three core questions they draw up are:

1 what is equity in health care?
2 equity of what?
3 what is financial equity?

I think that (1) and (3) are intertwined in that they both deal with equity in health *care*. We cannot achieve equity in health care delivery, which to me means 'equal access (or use) for equal need' if the financial contributions from current or future users are not established completely *independently* of their needs for health care. This corresponds with what Alan described as the egalitarian viewpoint in his guide through the ideological jungle (Williams, 1988a), whereby health care is being distributed according to *need* and financed according to *ability to pay*. Wagstaff and van Doorslaer (2000) distinguish between divorcing payment from utilisation (delivery), and divorcing payment from ability to pay (finance).

When healthcare finance is included as a non-earmarked tax, the level of financial equity depends on the level of progressivity in income taxation – an issue of fair taxation that lies in the Treasury. Hence, Aki and Paul's *third* core question – what is financial equity? – is essentially an issue that lies outside the Department of Health (at least in a UK and Norwegian context).

As to their *first* core question – what is equity in health care? – most authors emphasise the instrumental nature of equity in health *care*, as a precondition for achieving equity in health, which is the heart of their *second* core question.

DISCUSSION

My discussion can be summarised in a box:

	Equity	Fairness
Health care	I	II
Health	III	IV

I: Equity in health care – equal access (or use) for equal need

I will bypass the discussion on access versus utilisation, as both terms deal with equity in health *care*. For identical needs (same ill-health *and* same capacities to benefit), equity in health care means that people are equally entitled to, and are considered to have the same rights to, health care – completely independently of any non-medical characteristics of the recipients (e.g. most importantly income). This corresponds with the egalitarian camp in the jungle! In principle, the degree of various types of inequality in healthcare utilisation, or access, can be measured empirically, e.g. use of health care across social classes.

II: Fairness in health care – which types of inequalities are acceptable?

According to Elster (1992) 'the tasks of the major theories of justice can be stated as *justifying deviations from equality*'. What is a fair, acceptable – or just – type of inequality in health or health care then? This is not only an issue of an equity–efficiency trade-off, like a degree of inequality as expressed in social welfare function (SWF) weight. It also deals with the *reasons* behind an inequality.

Le Grand (1987) argues that some types of inequalities in healthcare use are not inequitable as they result from different choices or preferences. Following Le Grand's conception of *equality of choice sets*, those inequalities in health that emerge from an equal choice set (opportunities) are considered fair or acceptable.

In the textbook *Strained Mercy*, Evans (1984) holds that '"need" also carries significant ethical overtones; its allegation asserts an obligation on others . . . that someone *ought* to do something'. This leads me to question whether we feel the same obligation on others – completely independent of the *cause* of their needs? While we do have *mercy*, when and why is it *strained*?

To me, Le Grand's arguments and those of many other authors who suggest that people should be held responsible for their own health-related behaviour – particularly so if well-informed – deal with *fairness* rather than equity *per se*. Are people equally entitled, and are all needs equally worthy of collective funding?

My message here is simply that I think that – when we think of it – a large proportion of the reasons people give for *justifying deviations from equality* in access to health care deal with issues concerning the *causes* of the need for health care (*see* Dolan and Olsen 2001; Olsen *et al.*, 2003).

III: Equity in health – equity of which health stream?

As for Aki and Paul's second core question – equity of what? – their emphasis throughout the paper is on health, and more precisely *total health* measured by expected lifetime QALYs (ELQ) as the distribuendum. This is associated with the 'fair innings' argument: reduce inequalities in ELQ by distributing QALY gains to those with shortest ELQ.

While I agree with Aki and Paul – and Alan – that ELQ is the most important stream of health in which to reduce inequalities, there are other potentially relevant streams. I know Aki and Paul agree, and they have even written a paper, as well as a reply to Nord (2006), on this (Dolan and Tsuchiya, 2005, 2006). Two alternative streams of health that might be 'distribuendum candidates' are:

- *prospective health:* differences in individuals' no-treatment health profiles are important for both ethical and equity reasons: if QALY gains are distributed to the most severely ill, inequalities in prospective health are reduced

- *health gains:* an important equity issue deals with the degree to which there is diminishing social value of increasing QALYs gained (Olsen, 2000).

IV: Fairness in health – which types of inequalities in health are acceptable?

In the following I shall stick to ELQ as the most relevant stream in which to reduce inequalities in health. But which types of inequalities in ELQ do we find acceptable, or fair – and for which ethical justification?

Aki and Paul refer to Alan's survey (Williams, 1988b) in which he questions whether or not the societal value of a unit of health should be regarded as equal across all types of patients. In other words, while equity involves that 'a QALY is a QALY is a QALY', what Alan opened up here was to ask under which circumstances people might think that 'a QALY is *not* a QALY is *not* a QALY'. Interestingly, of the eight different 'discriminators' Alan used in this pilot survey, the one that most respondents would take into account was whether 'people who have taken care of their own health should get preference over those who haven't'. The other discriminators dealt with age, consequences on others (caring and financial), and deprivation (social class). Although the setting of the questionnaire was NHS priorities, and thus fairness in the distribution of health *care*, it appears that the issue Alan sought to explore was which patient characteristics respondents would discriminate for or against, i.e. weighting of health gain units.

Again, I think 'fairness in health' also deals with the ethical justifications we give for *accepting inequalities* in health, i.e. under which circumstances we would think that 'a QALY is *not* a QALY is *not* a QALY'.

Interestingly, in their SWF, Aki and Paul assign equal weight to the two groups 'where the assumption is that neither party is responsible for the differences in their lifetime health'. They seem to imply that it is fair to assign *un*equal weights had one party been more responsible than the other.

Furthermore, based on some preliminary surveys, Aki and Paul ask if it could be that the fair innings argument will work across social classes, but not across gender. This corresponds with results I got in a Norwegian survey where only 5.8% would assign more weight to the health of the group with shortest life expectancy when this was men versus women, while 24% would do so when it was the lowest social class. In the case of smokers versus non-smokers, among those who were prepared to discriminate, more of them opted for the group with *highest* life expectancy. Again, this highlights the importance of looking at the *cause* behind an inequality. As Aki and Paul also accept, it is not only the degree of inequality in ELQ that matters for the elicitation of subgroup weights in a SWF, but the characteristic of the subgroups.

POLICY IMPLICATIONS

There is sufficient evidence to prove immense inequalities in health – across gender, social classes, regions, etc. In my view, the two most crucial questions are:

1 for which subgroup characteristics do we consider inequalities to be most unfair?
2 which policy sector should be held responsible for reducing the unfair inequalities?

As to the first question, social class seems to be the answer. The ideology behind public health care was based on the view that inability to pay is an *unacceptable reason* for denying people access to health care.

I think the second question depends on whether the observed inequalities in health are caused by inequalities in access to health care. If the answer is *yes*, the responsibility clearly lies within the health sector, and the policy implication might be one of allocating relatively more healthcare resources to those groups with lowest ELQ, e.g. by expanding healthcare provision in socially deprived areas. If the answer is *no*, I think the health sector responsibility issue is not that obvious. If health inequalities are caused by systematic variations in the determinants of ill-health, one might argue that it is the relevant host sectors of these determinants (e.g. housing, work safety) that should be held responsible, rather than suggesting that it is the responsibility of the health sector to repair these inequalities.

Even if all current healthcare resources were allocated to the lower social classes, we might still not achieve complete equality in ELQ. However, *if* it turned out to be technically feasible to reduce inequalities in ELQ by a radical reallocation of NHS resources towards the lower social classes, such a health policy might still not be considered *fair*.

FURTHER RESEARCH PRIORITIES

First, concepts: Alan and Richard Cookson in their *Handbook of Health Economics* chapter (Williams and Cookson, 2000) held that in economics, '"fairness' is taken almost unthinkingly to mean *reducing inequalities*' (italics in original). As emphasised above, to me fairness has more connotations about which sorts of – and levels of – inequalities most people would consider acceptable. I think there is a need for some clarifications regarding what we mean by *fairness in health and health care*. Those who are prepared to explore this controversial issue of letting personal health responsibilities matter, might wish to consult Lake's book *Equality and Responsibility* (2001), which attempts to bring together ideas on equal distributions of goods with ideas on what people are responsible for.

Aki and Paul set out three main research directions. The first is more descriptive including 'the determinants of the variation of ELQ'. I would say 'the variation in the determinants of ELQ', and draw attention to a framework that I developed together with Paul (Dolan), Jeff Richardson and Paul Menzel (Olsen *et al.*, 2003). The causes, or determinants, of (ill-) health are of three types:

1 genetics (the biological lottery)
2 environment (the social lottery)
3 health-related lifestyle (explained by social conditioning and preferences).

These determinants are then located on a continuum with different degrees of individual control, and hence responsibility, for own health. My point is that while these three sets of determinants are analytically the same for all of us, there are huge variations in how they hit us, and hence impact on our health; e.g. the higher social classes have been luckier in the social lottery (or chosen a healthier environment, if you so prefer). I think that more *analytical* descriptive research on variations in the determinants of ELQ is needed – a prime example of which is the book edited by Bob Evans (1994), simply and neatly called *Why are Some People Healthy and Others not? The determinants of health of populations*. So, yes, this research direction is important – particularly if policy focused and evidence based.

Aki and Paul's second direction involves economic theory and empirical work related to a health-related social welfare function. This is where I perceive them to intend to be 'extending the Williams way'. Interestingly, within Alan and Richard Cookson's handbook taxonomy of 'Theories of equity in the distribution of health', Aki and Paul's type of SWF comes under the label 'non-linear and smooth'. Like most people, including economists, I find smooth curves much more appealing than linear or kinked ones, so I don't blame them! However, while I find iso-welfare curves nice in theory, I am pessimistic when it comes to measuring stable preferences in terms of people's willingness to forgo overall health for more equal distribution. Aki and Paul acknowledge the complications and ask: 'whether or not preferences elicited from the general public will be as well behaved as expected by theory?' I believe such preferences are extremely sensitive to framing and context, including other streams of health such as severity levels and the absolute magnitudes of health gains. However, I share Aki and Paul's interest in understanding the *reasons* that respondents give for their trade-offs, i.e. which types and levels of inequalities people consider to be fair.

The third research direction they outline is expanding into the economics of well-being. Well, it might well be a possible avenue for further work, particularly so if that is the interest of the researchers.

Then finally, I would like to thank Aki and Paul for a truly stimulating paper. I certainly think it has extended *my way* of thinking about equity and fairness in health and health care.

REFERENCES

Dolan P and Olsen JA (2001) Equity in health: the importance of different health streams. *Journal of Health Economics* **20**: 823–34.

Dolan P and Tsuchiya A (2005). Health priorities and public preferences: the relative importance of past health experience and future health prospects. *Journal of Health Economics* **24**: 703–14.

Dolan P and Tsuchiya A (2006) Severity of illness and priority setting: worrisome criticism of inconvenient finding? – A reply to Erik Nord. *Journal of Health Economics* **25**: 173–4.

Elster J (1992) *Local Justice: how institutions allocate scarce goods and necessary burdens.* New York: Russell Sage Foundation.

Evans RG (1984) *Strained Mercy: the economics of the Canadian health care.* Toronto: Butterworths.

Evans RG, Barer M and Marmor T (eds) (1994) *Why are Some People Healthy and Others not? The determinants of health of populations.* New York; A de Gruyter.

Kahneman D, Knetsch JL and Thaler R (1986) Fairness as a constraint on profit seeking: entitlement in the market. *American Economic Review* **76**: 728–41.

Lake C (2001) *Equality and Responsibility*. Oxford: Oxford University Press.

Le Grand J (1987) Equity, health and health care. *Social Justice Research* **1**: 257–74.

Nord E (2006) Severity of illness and priority setting: worrisome lack of discussion of surprising finding. *Journal of Health Economics* **25**: 170–2.

Olsen JA (2000) A note on eliciting distributive preferences for health. *Journal of Health Economics* **19**: 541–50.

Olsen JA, Richardson J, Dolan P and Menzel P (2003) The moral relevance of personal characteristics in setting health care priorities. *Social Science and Medicine* **57**: 1163–72.

Rawls JA (1958) Justice as fairness. *Philosophical Review* **67**: 164–94.

Wagstaff A and van Doerslaer E (2000) Equity in health care finance and delivery. In: Culyer AJ and Newhouse JP (eds) *Handbook of Health Economics.* Amsterdam: Elsevier, pp. 1803–62.

Williams A (1988a) Priority setting in public and private health care: a guide through the ideological jungle. *Journal of Health Economics* 7: 173–83.

Williams A (1988b) Ethics and efficiency in the provision of health care. In: Bell JM and Mendus S (eds) *Philosophy and Medical Welfare.* Cambridge; New York: Cambridge University Press, pp. 111–26.

Williams A and Cookson R (2000) Equity in health. In: Culyer AJ and Newhouse JP (eds) *Handbook of Health Economics.* Amsterdam: Elsevier, pp. 1863–910.

CHAPTER 10

Putting the 'Q' in QALYs

... Paul Kind

INTRODUCTION

The quantification of the benefits of healthcare interventions, their description and valuation form the central foundation for economic evaluation. For more than 30 years Alan Williams helped shape the development of thinking and practice in a field of enquiry that he once described as being 'not strictly speaking economics' (Williams, 1974), motivated in part by what he saw as the reluctance of other professional groups 'to plunge into the difficult territory of devising output measures for health care systems'. The quality-adjusted life year (QALY) represents one of the most elegant forms of such outcome measurement, combining information on '*both intensity and duration*'. The central role accorded to QALYs by today's analysts and decision makers bears witness to the leadership and perseverance of those who struggled with a technology that continues to provoke challenge.

The early mantra of 'a QALY is a QALY is a QALY' has given way to a more complex debate concerning issues of distribution, of equity and (paradoxically) monetary value. It is not the purpose of this paper to rehearse any of this material but rather to focus on the one issue that has remained at the heart of the QALY matter, namely the mechanism by which the quality-adjustment factor needed in computing QALYs is (and should be) established. Today we can turn for advice on such technical matters to any number of agencies (National Institute for Clinical Excellence (NICE), 2004), books (Gold *et al.*, 1996; Drummond *et al.*, 2005) or indeed health economists. It was not always so. Literature that is currently listed under the keyword 'quality of life' was referenced in the days of *Index Medicus* under the category of 'health status'. Neither was the combination of information on duration/survival and health status the exclusive creation of the health economist, with for example, well-years as a unit of measure being proposed by clinicians as the integral of health status over time (Grogono and Woodgate, 1971). The richness and diversity of today's research contrasts with the simplicity and single-mindedness of the work that predates it.

BACKGROUND AND EVOLUTION

At about the same time that interest in cost–benefit analysis was emerging in the 1960s, we can see the first serious attempts to address ways of measuring health status, although the focus was largely directed at the level of the population and relied principally on the use of mortality data. The influential contributions of Sanders (1964) and Sullivan (1966) continue to resonate today in the use of summary measures of population health (SMPH), and more generally in the concept of health-adjusted life expectancy (HALE). Assigning a year of life with no disability and a year of life with any disability a 'value' of 1 and 0 respectively, and combining this coding convention with actuarial life tables, it is possible to compute the years of life with or without disability. Disability-free life expectancy (DFLE) is of greatest interest to medical demographers and others concerned with an ageing population. It is not just that life expectancy is increasing, but of particular concern is whether the ill-health component is on average being compressed and delayed – do people enjoy relative improvements in survival without problems in young to middle age, only to have to face problems in later years? While the question itself may be interesting, it is the techniques applied to its investigation that are the focus of this paper, namely the convention applied to the description and valuation of health. The very mention of 'disability' can be highly provocative, especially in the context of the disability/impairment/handicap debate. The data used more recently to compute DFLE in the UK were derived from the limiting long-standing illness question contained in the General Household Survey question. Individuals who report any degree of limitation in the past two weeks and who have a chronic problem of any sort are categorised as 'disabled' and assigned an identical value of zero. All other individuals, regardless of their experience in the remainder of the year, share the value 1.

At about this time in the US, Fanshel and Bush (1970) published their seminal work describing a health status index for use in investigating changes in population health status engineered by health treatment. They noted with dismay the shortcomings of (then) current indicators based on mortality and the reliance on measures of activity rather than outcome.*

The model described for their index was hugely influential, leading directly to the Quality of Well Being (QWB) scale (Patrick *et al.*, 1973) and to related methodological research that was widely cited over the following decade. Set within their original paper are suggestions for obtaining values for functional states defined by any health status index. Their general procedure of choice

* The provision of health services is a $60 billion-a-year enterprise, yet no comparable industry spends so little on evaluating its own performance. More is known about the consumption of macaroni and corsets than the health status of the population.

BOX 10.1 THREE-DIMENSIONAL DESCRIPTIVE SYSTEM

Mobility

1(a) Ability to get in and out of bed and/or chair
1(b) Ability to negotiate a level surface
1(c) Ability to climb stairs
1(d) Ability to walk outdoors

Capacity for self-care

2(a) Ability to feed self
2(b) Ability to dress self
2(c) Ability to wash self
2(d) Ability to make a hot drink
2(e) Ability to cook a meal
2(f) Ability to light a fire
2(g) Ability to shop
2(h) Whether or not continent

Mental state

3(a) Intellectual processes – memory and orientation of person and place
3(b) Loneliness and desolation
3(c) Depression
3(d) Boredom
3(e) Motivation towards independence
3(f) Anxiety
3(g) Antisocial or self-harming behaviour

Source: Williams A (1974) Measuring the effectiveness of health care systems. *British Journal of Preventive and Social Medicine* **28**: 196–202. Reproduced with permission from the BMJ Publishing Group.

is that of paired comparisons (Thurstone, 1927) and they describe a range of variants based on weighting through equivalence in time, population and dysfunctional history. These correspond to the current techniques of time trade-off (TTO) and person trade-off (PTO).

First articulated in a paper co-authored with Culyer and Lavers (Culyer *et al.*, 1972), Williams described a health status classification system based on three 'divisions' – mobility, capacity for self-care and mental state as shown in Box 10.1 – which defined 64 possible health states. He observed that 'the major stumbling block at present is the absence of any widely used standardized descriptive categories of social functioning and that without these we cannot get off first base' (Williams, 1974). He foresaw a two-stage solution to the problem of measuring the (dis)benefits of health care which ideally would be expressed 'in monetary units commensurate with the relevant cost estimates'. Health states defined by a set of descriptive categories of the type proposed in Box 10.1 would be assigned index values on a scale of ill-health intensity. The 10-point scale he proposed was not dissimilar to that originally described by Karnofsky *et al.*, (1948) with endpoints 'normal' and 'dead' being valued as 0 and 10 respectively. The final step in the process was to attach money values to the index points, a process that he suggested might be undertaken using methods applied in constructing an index of the seriousness of crime (Sellin and Wolfgang, 1964).

At roughly the same time, Rachel Rosser was developing a separate descriptive classification system based on twin dimensions of disability and distress, divided into 8 and 4 levels respectively. This 8*4 system defined a total of 28 health states, since it was held that being unconscious (disability level 8) necessarily implied that there could be no distress. This simple generic classification had been designed using clinician focus groups. Initial attempts to associate a value with these 28 health states had involved the analysis of legal awards data determined in civil actions in English courts (Rosser and Watts, 1972). Judgements in these cases specifically dealt with the compensation awarded to plaintiffs in respect of loss of physical function (disability) and pain (distress). Rosser recognised an important limitation in this approach, not least being the metric itself, but also that other factors might be relevant in determining the value associated with different health states; these included the personal characteristics of those who made such value assignments – in particular, their age and current health status and exposure to those in poor health. Additionally, she identified the importance of framing effects including prognosis and the time spent in ill-health states. Using techniques imported from management science, Rosser conducted a series of interviews in which multiple valuation methods were used to elicit scores for disability/distress health states, including magnitude estimation, equivalence scaling and standard gamble procedures (Churchmann *et al.*, 1957). However, it was the magnitude estimation values derived from interviews with a convenience sample of 70 individuals with different current health experiences that formed the centrepiece of this work (Rosser and Kind, 1978). Following the publication of these values for disability/distress states and further analysis around the valuation of death (Kind and Rosser, 1980), it was Alan Williams who proposed the notion of transforming the original values so that they took on the anchor points of 1 for full health and 0 for dead. It is worth noting that more than half the health states occupy the value space between 0.9 and 1.0 (as can be seen in Table 10.1). The subsequent publication of a scale of health state values based on the transformed median magnitude estimation data (Kind *et al.*, 1982) ultimately proved to be something of a turning point, since it provided health economists, in the UK at least, with the first standardised generic measure with the capacity to compute QALY calculations using weights of domestic origin.

TABLE 10.1 MEDIAN DISABILITY/DISTRESS STATE VALUATIONS BASED ON MAGNITUDE ESTIMATION

Disability/distress	a	b	c	d
1	1.000	0.995	0.990	0.967
2	0.990	0.986	0.973	0.932
3	0.980	0.972	0.956	0.912
4	0.964	0.956	0.942	0.870
5	0.946	0.935	0.900	0.700
6	0.875	0.845	0.680	0.000
7	0.677	0.564	0.000	-1.486
8	-1.028			

Source: Kind P, Rosser RM and Williams A (1982) Valuation of quality of life: some psychometric evidence. In: Jones-Lee MW (ed.) *The Value of Life and Safety.* Collection of Papers presented at the Geneva Conference on The Value of Life and Safety held at the University of Geneva, 30 March to 1 April, 1981. By permission of the Geneva Association; Elsevier; and Professor Michael Jones-Lee. Distress scale: *a* (no distress) to *d* (severe distress); Disability scale: 1 (no disability) to 8 (unconscious).

Writing at about this time, Weinstein and Stason (1977) observed that although still controversial, methods for explicitly incorporating quality-of-life concerns into formal cost-effectiveness analyses were becoming more widely used and accepted. They went on to exemplify the mechanism by which the weighting system for such quality adjustment should be made, namely using standard gamble (SG) or TTO. A formal justification for the selection of 'utility' weights in this role in computing QALYs was not put forward in this paper (Pliskin *et al.*, (1980) appear to provide that methodological argument).

By the mid-1980s the ground had been prepared for a veritable explosion of research activity related to the science of quality-of-life measurement. Established generic measures included the QWB and the Sickness Impact Profile (SIP) (Bergner *et al.*, 1976) of US origin as well as the UK analogue, the Nottingham Health Profile (NHP) (Hunt *et al.*, 1985). In Finland, Harri Sintonen (1981) had developed the 15D and in Canada the Health Utilities Index (HUI) was in being (Torrance *et al.*, 1982). The long-form precursor to what became the SF-36 was already in place (Ware and Sherbourne, 1992). At York, researchers were concentrating on the issue of valuation in general, and values for the disability/distress states in particular. The use of magnitude estimation methods was not itself a concern, rather it was that the size and nature of Rosser's sample of respondents rendered questionable the status of the resulting value matrix as representative of social preferences. Efforts to replicate the original value set produced equivocal results (Gudex *et al.*, 1993).

In 1987 a group of researchers met in Rotterdam, at Alan Williams' behest, with the objective of exploring their common interest in the valuation of health.

The resulting network of researchers later became known as the EuroQoL group and continues to thrive as an international scientific community. The central question that interested its founding members survives to this day, namely how do values for health vary across countries (and to a lesser extent within population subgroups)? In order for the group to begin investigating this subject it required two things – a standardised method of describing health states and a single common method of valuing those health states. The first of these requirements was met by formulating a descriptive system initially based on six dimensions. This descriptive system was fairly rapidly modified after initial testing by merging two dimensions, yielding five: mobility, self-care, usual activities, pain/discomfort and anxiety/depression. Each dimension had three possible levels of response corresponding to no problem, some problem and extreme problem. In combination they formed a descriptive classification of 243 health states, to which two further states were added – unconscious and dead. The group selected visual analogue scaling (VAS) as its standard valuation method, primarily because the investigation of values in the general population was to be conducted using postal survey methods and VAS was regarded as 'simple' enough to be used in this context. So that all research teams utilised the same protocol for investigating values within the different countries then represented within the group, a standard valuation questionnaire was devised in which a set of 16 health states was presented. It was recognised that for most people the concept of valuing health would certainly be a novel experience and potentially somewhat challenging. To introduce both the descriptive system and the VAS task, respondents were first asked to assess their own health status. It rapidly became clear that this preliminary two-page segment of the valuation questionnaire was capable of generating information of independent significance. The 'simple' descriptive classification was shown to be responsive to differences in age, current health experience, social class, educational attainment, housing tenure and health behaviours; a similar pattern was demonstrated in the self-reported VAS data. This type of variation, which seemed to be consistently in evidence in the various surveys conducted by researchers in the formative days of the EuroQoL group, confirmed the view that EQ-5D (as it subsequently became termed) had legitimate value as a measure of health-related quality of life.

EQ-5D is probably the most widely used of a small set of generic index measures of health-related quality of life that are appropriate for application in cost–utility analysis. This set additionally includes HUI, 15D, AQLQ (Asthma Quality of Life Questionnaire), SF-6D and QWB. In the context of UK decision making, it has achieved particular salience as a result of guidance on technology assessment issued by NICE. As with all measures of this type, EQ-5D conforms to a general model used by instrument developers from Bush onwards, and consists of two discrete but linked components. First, a standard descriptive system is used to classify patients into one of a fixed set of health states. A value or weight is assigned to this health state from a previously established valuation set that forms the second component in this general model. It is the means whereby these values are elicited, that is the central issue that dominates research (and practice) in measuring health outcomes for economic evaluation. From the outset the EuroQoL group encouraged local experimentation around this issue by its research membership. The sole proviso was that whatever else was done, the 'standard' valuation task would be administered alongside any other variant. The Measurement and Valuation of Health (MVH) project at York had already tested a variety of valuation methods including TTO and SG, and had selected the former as the basis of a national UK population survey conducted in 1993. The survey led to the production of a set of (TTO) utility weights for EQ-5D health states, somewhat awkwardly labelled a 'tariff'. At the time, the MVH protocol/survey represented the most sophisticated attempt to capture social preferences, and since then has been adopted (and adapted) in a number of other countries where domestic national value sets have been established. The production of the MVH value sets (some 32 different sets were published as part of the final report) raised new problems that had not hitherto appeared to be significant (or intractable). The foremost of these remains that of formulating a method to interpolate values for health states not directly recorded as part of the survey protocol. The MVH survey was based on a subset of 45 health states selected from the total descriptive array of 245. The modelling/interpolation effort invested in the MVH data by the York team, and by the EuroQoL group more generally, was frankly enormous and the data continue to be the subject of analysis to this day. A similar enterprise conducted with the benefit of computer-based adaptive testing methods could generate data that mitigated this need. The asymmetry in protocols for valuing health states better or worse than dead, indeed the entire question of the valuation of 'dead', became apparent in the aftermath of the survey and remain significant issues. The mere fact that the MVH protocol incorporated a TTO task does not resolve the issue of what constitutes *the* appropriate method of eliciting such values. As yet there has been no significant comparison of such values with those derived from SG. Finally, the assumed invariance of values for EQ-5D health states needs to be confronted. This is part of the wider agenda of the generalisability of health state values that first brought the EuroQoL group together. Do values obtained from a UK population survey properly represent the social preferences of the citizens of other countries? Can 'utility' weights generated by TTO legitimately substitute for SG weights? Do such weights change over time? The research agenda remains substantial.

THE CURRENT STATE OF PLAY

So to what point does this long journey of discovery now bring us? Are we closer to realising the aspiration of those who initially set all this in motion? Of the enduring nature of the QALY itself there seems little doubt. A recent

International Society for Pharmacoeconomics and Outcomes Research (ISPOR) symposium heard from critics and practitioners alike that they envisaged its continued survival. It is the means by which we achieve the 'Q' in QALYs that is of most importance, and it is here that there seems to be the greatest variability of interpretation. The Washington Panel of Cost-effectiveness in Health and Medicine distinguished between two broad approaches to the assignment of preference weights to health states in computing QALYs: those based on expected utility theory and those derived from psychological or psychophysical scaling methods (Gold *et al.*, 1996). It was noted that 'the diversity in how preference weights are gathered markedly constrains the ability to credibly compare analyses where the effectiveness measure is presented in QALYs' (Gold *et al.*, 1996, p. 119). The panel recognised what they politely termed 'disagreement' as to the best measurement strategy. The existence of a 'correct' method 'depends in the first instance', they suggested, 'on whether there are theoretical reasons for adopting a particular approach' (Gold *et al.*, 1996, p. 118). They go on intriguingly to state that 'it is not clearly the case that incorporation of risk attitudes into the utilities that represent the "quality" dimension of QALYs is necessary for CEA [cost-effectiveness analysis] studies designed to inform resource allocation decisions' (Gold *et al.*, 1996, p. 118). This position differs somewhat from the stance taken by

Response method	Question framing: Certainty (values)	Question framing: Uncertainty (utilities)
Scaling	1 Rating scale Category scaling Visual analogue scale Ratio scale	2
Choice	3 Time trade-off Paired comparison Equivalence Person trade-off	4 Standard gamble

FIGURE 10.1 A classification of preference-elicitation methods. *Source:* Drummond MF *et al.* (2005) *Methods for the Economic Evaluation of Health Care Programmes* (3e). Oxford: Oxford University Press, Table 6.1, p. 143. By permission of Oxford University Press.

NICE. In favouring cost–utility analysis as a means of providing 'a comparative context for judging the relative value of health benefits from interventions in different disease areas', NICE accords equal status to SG utilities and TTO utilities (NICE, 2001). As shown in Table 10.2, the reference case model most recently espoused by NICE is specific in rejecting preferences derived using rating scales. In his definitive review, Torrance (1986) clearly sets out the subtle but important difference between (vNM (von-Neumann and Morgenstern)) utility and values. The former can only be generated via choice-based methods operating under conditions of *uncertainty*. Everything else (at best) falls into the second category. This distinction is reinforced in at least one leading textbook (*see* Figure 10.1) (Drummond *et al.*, 2005).

Despite this accumulation of expert opinion to the contrary, the literature is replete with reports in which researchers claim that 'utilities' may be generated using one of three methods: SG, TTO or rating scales. It would be naïve in the extreme to expect that all methods would yield convergent results, or that there might be a single transformation that would convert one metric into another. Weights based on rating scale methods typically avoid explicit reference to uncertainty and exchange, so that in the strictest sense it is hard to see a case for their use as a cardinal measure of utility. However such methods do entail an element of choice, albeit one that is more subtly embedded. Analytical methods that enable cardinal scales to be derived from ordinal data generated by rating scales, have long been recognised, but these do not extend to the rote application of a power transformation, so often used as the mechanism for smartening-up such data.

TABLE 10.2 THE NICE REFERENCE CASE

Element of health technology assessment	The reference case
Measure of health benefits	QALYs
Description of health states for calculation of QALYs	Health states described using a standardised and validated generic instrument (#5.5.3)
Method of preference elicitation for health-state valuation	Choice-based methods, for example time trade-off or standard gamble, not rating scale
Source of preference data	Representative sample of the general public

Source: National Institute for Clinical Excellence (2004) *Guide to the Methods of Technology Appraisal.* London: NICE. Available at: www.nice.org.uk Reproduced and adapted with permission.

The hard fact of the matter is that the two principal methods of utility elicitation yield different estimates. Weights derived using SG are known to differ systematically from corresponding weights derived using TTO (Read *et al.*, 1984). The reluctance to entertain even the smallest risk of death in order to forego any portion of life expectancy at all, to avoid remaining in an apparently minor dysfunctional health state is well known. In the face of such demonstrable failure of the 'standard' techniques, researchers continue to struggle to reconcile the differences in empirical data generated using these methods. Were a sustainable case to be made that supported the dominance of SG, then the issue of valuation method might be settled once and for all. However, as noted by Brazier *et al.* (1999) 'if there is doubt about the axioms of expected utility theory as they relate to health state valuations, as many commentators suggest, there can be no justification for SG as the reference method or "gold standard" for health state valuation'. Furthermore, the practical procedure of implementing SG is itself open to widespread local variation. For example, there are at least three methods for determining indifference points other than the 'standard' ping-pong (top-down, bottom-up and iterative division). These different strategies can and do yield different results, so that even the existence of a 'standard' form of SG remains problematic.

Of equal importance in seeking to justify exclusive reliance on utility weights for QALY computation is the difficulty in establishing that *any* given set of weights does indeed possess the 'utility' attribute. A straw poll conducted among a convenience sample of health economists yielded a consensus that the attribute is conferred by virtue of the *method* by which the weights were obtained. But in the absence of a standardised protocol for determining 'utility' weights, it is hard to subscribe to this interpretation. It is this circularity that further weakens the case for the 'utility-only' approach to QALY calculation. Supposing that we are presented with two sets of weights and told that one was generated by SG/TTO methods and the other was an ordered set of numbers generated by the RAND function in Excel. What test would be used to determine the 'utility' set?

In fact, fairly simple attributes are required of the quality-adjustment factor used to compute QALYs. Table 10.3 sets out those attributes for QALYs in NICE appraisals. Some properties are more critical than others. For example, it would be inconceivable to undertake any arithmetic without access to a quality-adjustment factor with an index format. Nor would it be acceptable if such a factor lacked cardinal properties. These first four attributes are strictly non-negotiable, and failure to conform with any of them should be regarded as an irrecoverable defect. There *may* be more scope for flexibility in respect of the last two attributes. Accepting an alternative reference source could lead to the recognition of (say) patient-based values or those generated in a non-UK setting. In this regard it should be noted that since the MVH A1 value set represents the preferences of a *national* sample of the UK population, it allows Scottish 'voters' to influence decisions made on behalf of the English when applied in NICE appraisals. Not only did the Scottish respondents in the 1993 survey report poorer health status in themselves, they tended to assign lower values to EQ-5D health states than did their English counterparts. The effects of this health analogue to the West Lothian question have been described elsewhere (Kind, 2005).

TABLE 10.3 ATTRIBUTES OF QUALITY-ADJUSTMENT FACTORS

Attributes of the instrument	Critical issue	Scope for flexibility
Generic descriptive system	X	Nil
Index format	X	Nil
Cardinal scale	X	Nil
0 (dead) to 1 (full health) metric	X	Nil
'Principled' weighting system	X	Limited
Weights derived from relevant population	X	Limited

Table 10.4 sets out different approaches for distinguishing between preference-elicitation procedures used in QALY calculations. If utility measurement is an absolute requirement and SG is recognised as being the definitive method of choice, then TTO might be treated as close second and all other procedures would be grouped together. If the uncertainty requirement were removed, this would make any choice-based method acceptable, arguably with category rating and VAS being relegated to the second tier. The relative strength of preference can at least be inferred from any of the methods listed in Table 10.4, and in this respect there appears to be no way of distinguishing between these alternatives. So, if QALYs can only legitimately be computed using vNM utilities, then SG appears to be the lead method, with TTO acting as a proxy. If a more relaxed interpretation of social preferences is accepted, then methods that do not strictly yield utilities could be accepted as quality-adjustment weights in QALY calculations.

TABLE 10.4 HIERARCHY OF PREFERENCE-ELICITATION PROCEDURES

	A: choice based under uncertainty	B: choice-based methods	C: preference elicitation
Standard gamble	1	1	1
Time trade-off	2	1	1
Category rating	3	2	1
Visual analogue scale	3	2	1
Conjoint methods	3	1	1
Paired comparisons	3	1	1
Magnitude estimation	3	1	1
Equivalence matching	3	1	1

It may be noted as an aside that the high scruples now aspired to by NICE did not always constitute an obstacle to the dissemination of economic evaluation. The Rosser–Kind index was accepted even though it was based on the preferences of a small convenience sample using magnitude estimation methods. Rosser's second-generation instrument, the Index of Health-related Quality of Life (IHQL), was based on a form of SG methodology that had never been the subject of peer-review scrutiny and made no claim to represent population preferences. Nevertheless both systems have been used in QALY computations published by UK health economists as part of the NICE appraisal process.

It seems as though mainstream health economics continues to endorse the view that 'utilities' constitute the only legitimate form of adjustment weight in QALYs. This view appears to arise through vestigial attachment to the need for a methodological foundation grounded in economics or at any rate in a contiguous discipline. This in turn gives rise to the questionable position in which any 'utility'-based method is deemed acceptable, despite the manifest failure of the classical theory that provides its source DNA and from which these derivatives are formed. This is a weak and fundamentally indefensible position from which to operate, reminiscent of the last throes of the Flat Earth Society in the early days of space flight. Of course we can always find a justification for why the theory does not quite work as a model of real-world behaviours – we may simply regret man's inability to conform to expected utility theory; or we may construct experiments that test alternative explanations for the behaviours that violate the classical theory. When challenged over the friable nature of the theory to which health economics is apparently wedded, the response seems to be that at least there is a theoretical underpinning, unlike the position in other disciplines that deal with similar issues and where theory is held to be absent.

THE WAY AHEAD

As practitioners in the field of health economics we can choose between two alternatives. We might take the view that social preferences needed for computing QALYs must be expressed in terms of utilities that are derived from a choice-based methodology linked to relevant theory. In this situation, it is likely that the method by which utilities are generated would simply follow as a logical progression from theory into practice. This fortunate state of affairs would be further complemented by a high degree of consensus in academic circles about the theoretical basis of such measurement and the practical ways of achieving it. Furthermore, novel techniques could be empirically tested against that existing standard as a mechanism for determining their suitability as substitutes. Alternatively, we might consider that social preferences *may* be expressed as utilities, but that this is not an *absolute* requirement. The value associated with a health state may be determined by any one of a larger set of methods, the only constraint being that it must produce a single index value on a scale that assigns a value of 0 and 1 to 'dead' and 'full health' respectively. Both alternatives leave us well short of a sustainable position. Since different procedures for preference measurement tend to generate different values for a given health state, it will require an extraordinary piece of good fortune to come up with a plausible explanation or a unifying theory that allows for transformation between competing value sets. It could be that a retreat into an exclusive utility-based approach has some merit, since this would reduce the range of candidate methods. However, it would still leave us some way short of an accepted (or acceptable) common method.

In the absence of a recognised standard, multiple measurement methods must be tolerated as having some claim to legitimacy. The occasional happy accidental convergence of results offers some comfort that perhaps the picture is less complicated than others would have us believe. Widely differing results give further support for the view that different methods necessarily yield divergent results. The usual response to such a multiplicity of choice is to take refuge in sensitivity analysis rather than attack the problem head on. Does it make any difference to the conclusions if we apply one set of values/utilities or another? If quality adjustment is such a problematic task, then, despite the theoretical niceties, is it imperative that it is always undertaken as part of any cost-effectiveness analysis? Recent attention given to this question suggests that in many studies, *quality adjustment had relatively little effect on the final cost-effectiveness ratio*. Its impact was important in moving ratios across a $50 000/QALY cost-effectiveness threshold in only some 20% of the investigated cases (Chapman *et al.*, 2004). Where quality adjustment was indicated, then low-level investment in collecting preference data – for example using *ad hoc* adjustments – may be sufficient. Accepting the luxury of this approach leads to the inescapable conclusion that the choice of preference-elicitation method is an irrelevancy, and that ultimately any number will do. One way of addressing this decline into darkness would be to revisit the requirements of the reference case. Were NICE technical guidance to stipulate that all cost–utility analysis should be based upon a single generic instrument scored using a standard set of weights (perhaps regardless of their pedigree), then many of the problems associated with variability in quality-of-life data would be overcome. At least then the variability in reporting health outcomes could be contained.

True, where one door opens another closes and it would have to be recognised that some clinical studies would lack data based on that standard. But that is precisely the situation that holds today.

So for now we are faced with a real world that remains free of a consensus over the means by which social preferences of the population should be established. One consequence of this *laissez-faire* approach is that it permits the use of utility weights that only remotely connect with the specifications demanded for NICE appraisals. At this point, what seems to be the narrow issue about how to measure social preferences assumes a broader and more fundamental importance. The worldly pragmatists argue that decisions about the cost-effectiveness of new treatments have to be made, that we cannot wait for perfect measures or analytical tools, that uncertainty is endemic, that qualms about quality are not restricted to quality-of-life data, that NICE's determinations are not based solely on the cost-effectiveness evidence. All these arguments carry some weight of course, but they need to be seen from the perspective of society as a whole, not just from that vantage point of health economics or the scientific research community. Key to the long-term sustainability of NICE-type moderation of new health technologies is the extent to which the public remains convinced of the probity of the process and its outcomes. Decisions that appear to rely heavily on technically opaque methods offer natural targets for those disadvantaged by those decisions. It is too easy to dismiss such reactions as being the expected consequences from the usual suspects. Those close to the quality-of-life technology and its application in cost–utility analysis have a responsibility to act in ways that are compatible with the discharge of their roles as both scientists and citizens. To ignore or conceal issues that bear on the process of analysis is to risk long-term consequences that could disadvantage us all.

Nearly half a century has past since Bush, Torrance, Rosser, Williams and others first took up the challenge of measuring health outcomes. In the intervening period, the research landscape has profoundly changed with a complexity today that might have been difficult to envisage in those early days. The academic discipline of health economics was spawned during this time, and with it the emergence of cost–utility analysis in health. Despite some 25 years of sustained enquiry this central question of how to value health in QALY calculations remains both topical and largely unresolved. Perhaps now would be a good time to free ourselves from the self-imposed straitjacket of utility.

REFERENCES

Bergner M, Bobbitt RA, Kressel S *et al.* (1976) The Sickness Impact Profile: conceptual formulation and methodology for the development of a health status measure. *International Journal of Health Services* **6**: 393–415.

Brazier J, Deverill M, Green C *et al.* (1999) A review of the use of health status measures in economic evaluation. *Health Technology Assessment* **3**: 1–164.

Chapman RH, Berger M, Weinstein MC *et al.* (2004) When does quality-adjusting life years matter in cost-effectiveness analysis? *Health Economics* **13**: 429–36.

Churchmann CW, Ackoff RL and Arnoff E (1957) *Introduction to Operations Research.* New York: Wiley.

Culyer AJ, Lavers, RJ and Williams A (1972) Health indicators. In: Shonfield A and Shaw S (eds) *Social Indicators and Social Policy*. London: Heinemann, pp. 94–118.

Drummond MF, O'Brien B, Stoddart GL and Torrance GW (2005) *Methods for the Economic Evaluation of Health Care Programmes* (3e). Oxford: Oxford University Press.

Fanshel S and Bush JW (1970) A health-status index and its application to health-services outcomes. *Operations Research* **18**: 1021–66.

Gold MR, Patrick DL, Torrance GW *et al.* (1996) Identifying and valuing outcomes.

In: Gold MR, Russell LB and Weinstein MC (eds) *Cost-effectiveness in Health and Medicine*. New York: Oxford University Press, pp. 82–134.

Grogono AW and Woodgate DJ (1971) Index for measuring health. *Lancet* **2**: 1024–6.

Gudex C, Kind P, van Dalen H *et al.* (1993) *Comparing Scaling Methods for Health State Valuations: Rosser revisited. CHE Discussion Paper No.107.* York: University of York.

Hunt SM, McEwen J and McKenna SP (1985) Measuring health status: a new tool for clinicians and epidemiologists. *Journal of the Royal College of General Practitioners* **35**: 185–8.

Karnofsky DA, Abenmann WH, Craver LF and Burchenal JH. (1948) The use of nitrogen mustards in the palliative treatment of carcinoma. *Cancer* **1**: 634–56.

Kind P (2005) *The West Lothian Question – should Scottish 'voters' be included when valuing EQ-5D health states in England?* Proceedings of the EuroQoL Group Scientific 22nd Annual Plenary Meeting, Oslo, 8–10 September 2005.

Kind P and Rosser RM (1980) Death and dying: scaling of death for health status indices. In: Barber B, Gremy F, Überla K (eds) *Lecture Notes on Medical Informatics* **5**: 28–36. Berlin: Springer-Verlag.

Kind P, Rosser RM and Williams A (1982) Valuation of quality of life: some psychometric evidence. In: Jones-Lee MW (ed.) *The Value of Life and Safety*. Collection of Papers presented at the Geneva Conference on The Value of Life and Safety held at the University of Geneva, 30 March to 1 April, 1981. Amsterdam: North-Holland Publishing Company, pp. 159–70.

National Institute for Clinical Excellence (2001) *Guidance for Manufacturers and Sponsors: Technology Appraisals Process Series No. 5*. London: National Institute for Clinical Excellence.

National Institute for Clinical Excellence (2004) *Guide to the Methods of Technology Appraisal*. London: National Institute for Clinical Excellence.

Patrick DL, Bush JW and Chen MM (1973) Methods for measuring levels of well-being for a health status index. *Health Services Research* **8**: 228–45.

Pliskin S, Shepard DS and Weinstein MC (1980) Utility functions for life years and health status. *Operations Research* **28**: 206–24.

Read JL, Quinn RJ, Berwick DM, Fineberg HV and Weinstein MC (1984) Preferences for health outcomes. Comparison of assessment methods. *Medical Decision Making* **4**: 315–29.

Rosser RM and Kind P (1978) A scale of valuations of states of illness: is there a social consensus? *International Journal of Epidemiology* **7**: 347–58.

Rosser RM and Watts VC (1972) The measurement of hospital output. *International Journal of Epidemiology* **1**: 361–8.

Sanders BS (1964) Measuring community health levels. *American Journal of Public Health* **54**: 1063–70.

Sellin T and Wolfgang ME (1964) *The Measurement of Delinquency*. New York: Wiley.

Sintonen H (1981) An approach to measuring and valuing health states. *Social Science and Medicine* **15**: 55–65.

Sullivan DF (1966) *Conceptual Problems in Developing an Index of Health*. Washington: Office of Health Statistics Analysis, Department of Health, Education and Welfare.

Thurstone LL (1927) The method of paired comparisons for social values. *Journal of Abnormal Psychology* **21**: 384–400.

Torrance GW (1986) Measurement of health state utilities for economic appraisal: a review. *Journal of Health Economics* **5**: 1–30.

Torrance GW, Boyle MH and Horwood SP (1982) Application of multiattribute utility theory to measure social preferences for health states. *Operations Research* **30**: 1043–69.

Ware JE and Sherbourne CD (1992) The MOS 36-item short form health status survey (SF-36) I: Conceptual framework and item selection. *Medical Care* **30**: 473–83.

Weinstein, MC and Stason WB (1977) Foundations of cost-effectiveness analysis for health and medical practices. *New England Journal of Medicine* **296**: 716–21.

Williams A (1974) Measuring the effectiveness of health care systems. *British Journal of Preventive and Social Medicine* **28**: 196–202.

CHAPTER 11

Discussion of Paul Kind's paper: 'Putting the "Q" in QALYs'

... Ben van Hout

INTRODUCTION

In the same way as Kind's paper describes the background behind the development of the QALY, it may be useful to provide some historical notes from a slightly different perspective.

At the end of the 1980s, Dutch policy makers were searching for ways to limit the growth of expenditure on health care. Reports were published with titles such as 'Limits to growth' (of the insurance package), and a national debate was fought over 'Dunning's filter' (named after a professor of cardiology), a system devised to stop inefficient, costly and unnecessary technologies from receiving reimbursement. All this activity implied that choices had to be made about funding health care: choices about what should and should not be reimbursed and for whom and under what conditions. Moreover, the mechanisms by which such choices were made needed to be transparent, because explicit choices are open to debate. At the same time, the Dutch government initiated a number of large studies, fashionably called 'technology assessments', to evaluate heart transplantation, liver transplantation and *in vitro* fertilisation. At the centre of these studies was the assessment of costs and effects. In those days, methods to assess the cost-effectiveness of public programmes could be found in the text books of Mishan (1982), Dasgupta and Pearce (1978) and Sugden and Williams (1978). They offered researchers a frame of reference in which changes were assessed using concepts such as 'opportunity costs' 'equivalent variation' and 'compensating variation'.

'Compensating variation' refers to the amount of money that one has to give a person to make him as happy after a change as he was before that change. In 1978, Broome pointed out that it is somewhat difficult to establish the amount of money needed to make dead people as happy as when they were alive and that 'the attempt to value life in terms of money is more or less doomed to failure' (Broome, 1978). A lively debate followed in which Alan Williams (Williams, 1979) was one of several famous economists (Jones-Lee, 1979; Mishan, 1981) who wrote replies to Broome's critique. Mishan's offer to help 'to clear the cobwebs from his [Broome's] mind and to restore perspective' illustrates that the economists were not persuaded by Broome's arguments. However, an atmosphere was created in which it seemed politically incorrect to value the effects of medical treatments in monetary terms. It is possible that this catalysed Alan Williams's efforts to try to develop a less controversial measure that could be used without the accusation of applying a single-minded, short-sighted, internally inconsistent pseudo-science.

THE EUROQOL GROUP

Researchers in York were not the only ones searching for a scale to enable the comparison of treatment effects in different therapeutic areas for the sole purpose of the application in economic analyses. Dutch researchers were facing the same questions, and the contact between York and Rotterdam was also mediated via Brunel where Martin Buxton was sharing similar experiences concerning the evaluation of heart and liver transplantation. In my view, the central problem posed by the founding members of the EuroQol group was not – as Kind states – whether values for health differ between countries, but rather an economic one: to devise a metric that could be used in economic evaluations that would facilitate the decision-making process for policy makers. The presence of psychologists in the group was – from the perspective of the economists – instrumental. They didn't share the same problem, but they did hold most of the solution. And while the landmark publication about the cost-effectiveness of bypass surgery (Williams, 1985) could never have been written without the work of Rosser and Kind, it should be noted that QALYs have always been designed as a solution to an economic problem: the allocation of scarce resources within health care based on the assessment of costs and effects.

QALY

The 'best' way to derive the values which inform the Q element of the QALY may remain the subject of debate for many years to come. This process may be prolonged if the same system is also expected to be used for decisions other than those to do with resource allocation. One reason for this is that it is often very unclear what people mean by 'best'. When the goal is to support decision making it is indeed *the extent to which the public remains convinced of the probity of the process and its outcomes*. And indeed, when harsh decisions are taken there will always be groups who are disadvantaged and who will challenge the methods that were used. However, as Kind notes, the occasions where QALY calculations have been crucial, are limited. From a decision maker's perspective, the calculation of the balance between cost and effects is like a diagnostic test. Sometimes an intervention is clearly not cost-effective, sometimes it clearly is cost-effective but often one has to do some additional work. This may be in the form of additional research, additional considerations or both. The balance between costs and effects is assessed to define whether we are in a white, a black or in a grey area. Thresholds, such as say £30 000 per QALY gained, may be a trigger for doubts and for further thoughts. Such doubts are usually more about whether the threshold is correct, whether there are sufficient numbers of patients, whether the trial data are generalisable or whether there should be certain restrictions, than about the valuation technique used to calculate the QALY weights. This leads to a more pragmatic approach, or what may be termed 'a decision-maker's approach'. Such a view is probably quite close to the one held by Alan Williams, and one wonders whether he was one of the purist health economists Kind refers to. Alan's decisions to transform the values under 0 to a limit of –1, and to use means instead of medians (something he later seemed to regret), suggested that he was not. For him, political acceptability seemed to score more highly than scientific rigour. Additionally, Alan was also very aware of Joan Robinson's view that 'Utility is a metaphysical concept of impregnable circularity; utility is the quality in commodities that makes individuals want to buy them, and the fact that individuals want to buy them shows that they have utility' (Robinson, 1962). In other words 'real economists' know that they can't measure utility, but can only derive it by observing real behaviour, something that in health care is rarely done. Instead, economists are asked to 'prescribe' what a society *should* decide rather than 'describe' what 'typical' people *do* decide. Moreover, they do not really have any experience with doing this. Given that the whole question is about choices, and given that it has to be done on a collective basis, it may be best to derive the answers by asking people to decide in imaginary situations. Whatever the method, the concept of choice is eminently present.

VALUATION METHODS

The fact that decision makers might be less worried about the theoretical underpinnings of their value sets than purist economists (whoever these are) does not mean that they do not have any preferences about the ideal attributes for a value set. A good start might be a scale that puts 1 at perfect health, dead at 0, non-perfect states that are better than dead between 0 and 1, and states worse than dead below 0. Additionally, the scale would ideally have cardinal properties such that a year in a state of 0.50 is about equal to two years in 0.25. The latter is a harsh requirement whatever the technique used to derive the scale. As Kind points out, time trade-off and standard gamble seem to be the preferred methods, with visual analogue scaling, category rating and some discrete choice models following at a respectable distance. According to Kind, this distance was created by NICE and not by theory. Unfortunately, nobody will ever know whether he is right or wrong. There is no gold standard, and the fact that discrete choice models are often used in other areas does not mean that they give the right scale, either in their existing applications or in health.

When the aim is to value and compare a number of life years gained in states *x*, *y* and *z*, TTO seems to be the method that most closely reflects the question, in that it explicitly asks for the value of a given number of years in these health states. In contrast, standard gamble requires one to imagine a risk-taking situation. Visual analogue scaling and category rating only have an implicit choice element. Furthermore, all the discrete-choice methods need additional heroic assumptions before being able to derive a meaningful scale.

Research has shown that each method produces a slightly different scale. All methods seem to have their pros and cons. In order to decide whether one is better than any other, one has to define 'better'. Better – in light of the use in economic evaluations (the beginning of the EuroQol group) should be concerned with whether a different method would lead to decisions that better reflect what the majority of society prefers. At this point one may also wonder whether a different method would lead to any change in the decisions that are currently being taken. In addition, the decisions have to be defended in public and, in the absence of a gold standard, basing them on a method that seems intuitively closest to the original question seems as good as any other.

There are a number of different value functions for EQ-5D available, based on different sets of data. The so called 'A1 tariff', as derived from the TTO questions in the MVH study, is probably most often used. This is not only in the UK but also in the Netherlands where the logical preference for a Dutch tariff does not always prevail. The perceived effect on the probability of an international publication often outweighs any other argument. Indeed it is questionable whether using other value sets leads to different orderings of therapies which should be reimbursed. And indeed it may be suggested – as Kind does – that it is a scientific duty to keep on checking whether we are still on the right path. However, there is also something of a scientific duty to focus one's brain-power where it is most needed. This may be what Claxton (1999) refers to when considering the value of perfect information. And one may wonder whether Alan Williams wasn't one of the first to apply this concept when allocating his research activities away from QALYs, towards other issues such as those about equity weights?

THE GOLD STANDARD

Each valuation method has its own advantages and disadvantages, and one may never get to a gold standard in the sense of a perfect diagnostic test. The word 'gold standard' however may apply in its more traditional meaning. Just as in the late 19th century gold was arbitrarily chosen above silver after years of attempts to maintain a bimetallic standard, TTO might just be accepted as the standard. Maybe one should just accept that Alan Williams – or the MVH study for that matter – has defined TTO as the gold standard, just like the Germans decided in favour of gold when they wanted to be paid after the 100-year war.

ABOUT TTO

That TTO may be identified as the 'reasonable' Alan Williams way and thus as the way to go, does not imply that it is beyond improvement. For example TTO was used to estimate the impact of various degrees of erectile dysfunction and estimated the QALY weight for a complete dysfunctional state at 0.74 (Stolk *et al.*, 2000). This led to a very favourable cost-effectiveness ratio for Viagra. But the Dutch government decided not to reimburse it. This suggests that the valuation was not accepted to really reflect the disease burden. And indeed, taking a chance of 25% to die on an operating table, or to be in coma for almost two days a week just to be perfectly 'erectile ready' for the rest of the week, may seem rather high. This is especially so considering that medications that have to be injected into the penis – and that offer effective relief of the problem – are hardly ever used. This type of revealed preference suggests that maybe this isn't as serious a health problem as Stolk's work implies.

Does this study mean that we should use a different method to TTO? Not necessarily, but is does suggest that maybe one should be careful applying TTO in a disease-specific context.

Defining TTO as the gold standard does not mean that one should stop exploring alternatives. However, it would be foolish not to anchor that work within the rich experience that is already available. Additionally, it would be rather foolish to step away from the face-validity that TTO brings with it. Any discrete-choice study aiming to establish value sets could be improved if informed by TTO values for a number of the states being evaluated. Analyses are needed in which times are traded off without using 'perfect health' as a comparator. Additionally, a deeper understanding of the values elicited using TTO is needed. The observation that respondents especially disagree about the positioning of 'death' (Macran and Kind, 2001) warrants further research.

ABOUT ALAN WILLIAMS

I think that knowing Alan Williams personally – talking to him at conferences – increased my scientific 'street cred' among other Dutch researchers. Knowing Alan was 'cool'. Moreover he has helped us, less talented health economists, so often. Whenever some ethicist stood up to challenge the fruits of our research, he was the first to take up the challenge and did so with a flair that many can only aspire to ever reach. He led an international battle, not just a personal or a UK one.

Alan Williams made an impact on many, and those who met him or read his work will easily remember him. There are parts of the world where one is not really dead as long as one is still remembered. This may imply that one is 'more dead' when remembered by only one person than when remembered by thousands; perhaps this might be scored on a type of 'scale', measuring how much someone lives on in other people's memories. On this scale – assuming that health economists count too – he might be close to being alive. I like that thought.

ACKNOWLEDGEMENTS

I would like to thank Susan Macran for very helpful comments.

REFERENCES

Broome J (1978) Trying to value a life *Journal of Public Economics* **9**: 91–100.

Broome J (1979) Trying to value a life; a reply. *Journal of Public Economics* **12**: 259–62.

Claxton K (1999) The irrelevance of inference: a decision-making approach to the stochastic evaluation of health care technologies. *Journal of Health Economics* **3**: 341–64.

Dasgupta AK and Pearce DW (1978) *Cost–benefit Analysis: theory and practice*. London: Macmillan.

Jones-Lee MW (1979) Trying to value a life – why Broome does not sweep clean. *Journal of Public Economics* **12**: 249–56.

Macran S and Kind P (2001) 'Death' and the valuation of health-related quality of life. *Medical Care* **39**: 217–22.

Mishan EJ (1981) The value of trying to value a life. *Journal of Public Economics* **15**: 133–7.

Mishan EJ (1982) *Cost–benefit Analysis*. London: Allen and Unwin.

Robinson J (1962) *Economic Philosophy*. London: Penguin.

Stolk EA, Van Busschbach J, Caffa M, Meuleman EJH and Rutten FFH (2000) Cost utility analysis of sildenafil compared with papaverine-phentolamine injections, *British Medical Journal* **320**:1165–8.

Sudgen R and Williams A (1978) *The Principles of Practical Cost–benefit Analysis*, Oxford: Oxford University Press.

Williams A (1979) Note on trying to value a life. *Journal of Public Economics* **12**: 257–8.

Williams A (1985) Economics of coronary artery bypass grafting. *British Medical Journal* **291**: 326–9.

CHAPTER 12

The measurement and valuation of public safety

... Paul Dolan and Aki Tsuchiya

INTRODUCTION

Policy makers strive to allocate limited public resources to where they will do the most good; that is, where the use of resources strikes the best balance between efficiency and equity. Determining an efficient allocation may be informed by the results of economic appraisals, which measure and quantify the costs and benefits of alternative allocation decisions. The UK Treasury *Green Book* (HM Treasury, 2003) recommends that, where possible, costs and benefits are expressed in monetary terms. The notable exception is health where benefits are expressed in terms of quality-adjusted life years (QALYs) (owing much to the work of Alan Williams, of course). This paper considers how the intangible losses from crime and the fear of crime can be measured and valued in ways that allow for the economic appraisal of interventions that seek to reduce crime and/or its impact. We consider how monetary valuations can be obtained and the possibility of developing what Alan referred to as a 'SALY' – a security-adjusted life year.

In fact, Alan first thought about crime in the late 1960s when he was seconded to the Treasury, and then to the Home Office, where he met Vincent Watts. Vincent was working on the ideas of US criminologists Thorsten Sellin and Marvin Wolfgang on quantifying the seriousness of delinquent behaviour, based on how members of the public perceived it. Shortly after, Alan was trying to work out a method of quantifying the seriousness of ill-health, so he contacted Vincent Watts to see if the criminologists' methodology could be applied in the area of health. This led Alan to Vincent's wife, Rachel Rosser, who, together with Paul Kind, was doing exactly that. So, the ideas from criminology were applied to health and we are applying the developments in the valuation of health back to crime (see Williams (2005) for this historical circle).

There is now interest in the Home Office in valuing the intangible losses from crime, i.e. the difficult-to-quantify losses arising from the emotional and physical effects of crime. The most recent version of the economic and social costs of crime published by the Home Office (Dubourg *et al.*, 2005) includes some of the direct costs of crime (such as direct costs to the criminal justice system, the treatment of health losses and indirect costs due to productivity losses), as well as estimates of the intangible victim costs of crime and the fear of crime based upon values we estimated using a QALY-type approach (Dolan *et al.*, 2005; Dolan and Peasgood, 2006). However, those estimates were based on poor-quality data and a number of rather heroic assumptions, and this paper considers ways in which more robust estimates of the losses in well-being from actual and anticipated criminal victimisation could be generated.

As with any valuation exercise, there are questions about *what* is to be valued and *how* it is to be valued. The simplest thing to value would be categories of crime (robbery, burglary etc.), without describing or valuing the specific consequences for well-being of those crimes. This has the advantage that data on categories of crime are routinely collected by the police and in the British Crime Survey (BCS). However, these categories are very broad and there is no such thing as a 'typical' burglary, for example (Semmens, 2004). In addition, it is virtually impossible to attribute particular fears to particular crimes. Furthermore, as in the valuation of health, naming the label associated with the medical or criminal cause (e.g. 'cancer' or 'robbery') will allow respondents to bring all sorts of theories and imaginations of their own to the evaluation exercise that are beyond the control of researchers, starting from what they think causes these problems (e.g. 'smoking' or 'provocation') to what happens to victims (e.g. 'side-effects of chemotherapy' or 'severe depression').

Alternatively, we can think of crime and the fear of crime as impacting upon important (and comparable) attributes of our well-being. This is the approach adopted in this paper. The advantage of viewing the effects of crime and the fear of crime in this way means that it will be possible to compare losses resulting from actual victimisation with losses that occur from the anticipation of victimisation. However, as we shall see in the next section, we know surprisingly little about the losses in well-being that result from criminal victimisation, as very few studies have systematically traced the experiences of the victims of crime, and we know even less about how the fear of crime impacts upon well-being. Given the paucity of any reliable data in relation to the type and extent of the losses in well-being arising from criminal victimisation and fear, there is an urgent need for studies of the long-term consequences of crime.

In order to relate 'epidemiological' data to valuation data, it is desirable to generate a classification system that allows the different attributes of well-being that are affected by crime to be combined into overall 'crime states', and we discuss what such a classification system might look like in the next section of this chapter. This, of course, has many parallels with the work into 'health states' in the last 20 years, which has seen the development of a number of generic health-state classification systems designed to allow the value of each state to be expressed on a single index scale. It could be that we should simply use one of the existing health measures (e.g. the EQ-5D) in a crime context, which would have the great advantage of allowing for cross-sectoral comparisons.

Unfortunately, as we shall also see in the next section, there are important differences between well-being losses from crime and those from ill-health. Moreover, the losses in well-being from a crime are caused by the wilful intent of the perpetrator (unlike accidents, where injuries may still be caused by others, but not intentionally). This intent to cause harm can result in the victim experiencing losses in well-being when there are no obvious health effects. Such considerations might result in there being a 'crime premium' associated with criminal victimisation as compared to injuries and psychological trauma in other contexts (Dolan *et al.*, 2005).

In the third section of this chapter, where much of the material is taken from Dolan *et al.* (2007) and where we are grateful to our co-authors Ann Netten and Joanna Shapland, we consider different ways of generating valuations for these crime states. We focus on methods that are preference based; that is, the well-being associated with different states of world is inferred from people's preferences over those states. As an alternative to preference-based methods, economists have begun valuing non-market goods by considering the effects on an individual's subjective well-being (SWB) of income and a non-market good and then estimating the required income compensation that would hold SWB constant following a change in the non-market good (Clark and Oswald, 2002). We do not consider this method further here (*see* Dolan and Peasgood (2006) for a critique of this method and a comparison with WTP).

Economists would typically prefer to infer monetary values from observing consumer behaviour (Atkinson *et al.*, 2004). If we had information about the demand for goods that are intended to reduce the likelihood of being a victim, it might be theoretically possible to tease out the component attributable to preventing the intangible consequences. However, even if we had good data on, say, the demand for burglar alarms, it would be a daunting task to break this down into its component parts. Another possibility is to try to see how the price of accommodation varies between different neighbourhoods with different characteristics, but there are so many factors that may affect the way that property prices vary from one neighbourhood to another that it is difficult to make accurate and robust attributions to any one of them, such as the number of crimes of a particular type. As a result, there is a shortage of useful revealed preference data about the values of preventing the intangible consequences of crime (Lynch and Rasmussen, 2001).

As a result, 'stated preference' methods have been developed, which elicit monetary values through hypothetical choices presented to respondents. In this context, this would involve asking respondents to state their maximum willingness to pay (WTP) for a change in well-being from one crime state to another. We discuss the possibility of eliciting values using WTP but, given some serious problems with the methodology, there are doubts about its suitability. We go on to consider methods developed by health economists to allow the calculation of QALYs, and suggest that data generated by a ranking exercise might represent a better way forward.

DESCRIBING THE INTANGIBLE LOSSES FROM CRIME AND THE FEAR OF CRIME

The best large-scale evidence on criminal victimisation in the UK comes from data collected as part of the BCS, which now consists of over 50 000 interviews with adults in the UK every year. The BCS reports physical injuries resulting from violent crime such as scratches, cuts, broken nose, chipped teeth etc. However, it does not indicate whether or not the injury received medical attention from a doctor, so the seriousness of the injury is not easily determined. The BCS also investigates the emotional impact of crime by asking questions about which type of emotional reactions were experienced as a result of being victimised. However, it is difficult to make comparisons across waves where the list of possible reactions changes. In addition, the BCS gives no indication of the frequency or intensity of each emotional reaction, and does not even ask how long ago the incident took place, which could be anything from a day to a year ago. What is needed, of course, is longitudinal studies.

Most of the longitudinal studies of victims of crime took place in the 1970s and 1980s and did not use general population samples (e.g. Shapland *et al.*, 1985). For these reasons, it is doubtful whether the results are sufficiently generalisable. Research by Denkers and Winkel (1997) is the only recent general population longitudinal study in Europe. They found that victims of crime systematically reported lower levels of well-being than non-victims (less satisfied with life, less positive affect, perceiving the world as less benevolent and themselves as less worthy) and, to some extent, higher levels of feeling vulnerable to victimisation (being afraid of crime, people or situations, crime having a greater potential negative impact). However, victims were also less happy than non-victims before the offence (suggesting that those who are less happy have a higher risk of victimisation), so not all the resulting greater unhappiness can be attributed to being a victim of crime.

The intangible losses from the fear of crime are also difficult to define, not least because the fear of crime is itself a nebulous concept (Hale, 1995). A general concern with fear-of-crime surveys is that they pick up a whole host of things, including emotions that are quite distinct from risk and fear, such as anger (Ditton *et al.*, 1999), and fear and anxieties caused by non-crime activities which people are unhappy about in their environment (Bannister and Fyfe, 2001). In this paper, we define the 'fear of crime' as all the intangible losses in anticipation of possible victimisation (Dolan and Peasgood, 2006).

The prominence given to the fear in criminology contrasts with the relative lack of prominence given to the 'fear of illness' in the evaluation of most healthcare technologies. We do not have time or space to go into this issue in any detail here, but you might like to ponder why a comprehensive economic evaluation of an intervention should not take full account of any changes in the frequency, intensity or duration of fear that an individual experiences as a result of that intervention. As an example, in its cost–benefit analysis of the acceptable defect rate in medical gloves, the Food and Drug Administration (FDA) in the US attached a monetary value to the reduced fear that individuals may experience from lower defect rates (see Adler, 2004).

As with criminal victimisation, there is very little longitudinal evidence in relation to the fear of crime, so it is difficult to determine its relationship (if any) with actual victimisation and its cumulative effects. What seems clear from an accumulation of cross-sectional evidence, though, is that victimisation does not, in itself, explain fear (Semmens, 2004). Indeed, victimisation may prompt reactions to crime that actually mediate fear (Winkel, 1998). Perhaps the most useful study for estimating the overall emotional losses from the fear of crime was carried out by Farrall and Gadd (2004), in which a general population sample were asked 'In the past year have you ever felt fearful about becoming a victim of crime?'. Those who respond positively were asked 'How frequently have you felt like this in the past year', and also asked 'On the last occasion, how fearful did you feel?' (with response categories of 'not very fearful', 'a little bit', 'quite fearful', and 'very fearful'). However, the time period specified will influence how respondents interpret the questions asked of them. For example, Winkielman *et al.* (1998) asked respondents about how much anger they had experienced over time frames of either one week or one year. People reported large amounts of anger for the week compared to what would be expected for a year if we extrapolated from the weekly reports to a full year.

However, the situation is not entirely hopeless. In their excellent review, Shapland and Hall (2004) provide a list of the effects commonly found in the criminological literature and this list, with some slight modifications, is given below:

1 initial shock and guilt at having become the victim of crime
2 physical injury, including permanent incapacity in a small number of cases
3 psychological effects, including fear, anger and depression, which, for some, may turn into longer-term depressive effects including sleeplessness and anxiety and, occasionally, into post-traumatic stress disorder (PTSD)
4 behavioural effects, involving changes to the victim's lifestyle, normally to avoid the situation or context in which the offence occurred
5 a loss of autonomy and increased vulnerability
6 a loss of trust/faith in society, particularly in the local community or in relation to the social group or place where the offence occurred.

The effects of the fear of crime would appear to be similar to the effects of criminal victimisation itself. For example, fearful people may modify their behaviour, e.g. by not engaging in pleasurable activities as much as they would like (walking the dog, going to the pub etc) or by undertaking additional security measures, such as locking windows and doors, which have an opportunity cost in terms of time. Or they may change their views about society, or feel vulnerable. The psychological losses will be similar too, ranging from affective reactions to more cognitive assessments of the likelihood of victimisation (Dolan and Peasgood, 2006).

Against this background, we have developed the preliminary descriptive system shown in the Appendix to this chapter. We have recently begun asking members of the general public about the face validity of this measure, and early results are encouraging (although there have been some questions about whether 'no constraints on behaviour' is really such a good thing). This descriptive system generates $4^5 = 1024$ possible outcomes. A six-dimension system could also be explored, where one of the dimensions could be monetary; this would allow for the direct estimation of monetary values, as discussed in the next section.

VALUING THOSE LOSSES

Monetary valuations

An ideal stated-preference study would give information about the current baseline risks of experiencing particular outcomes and encourage respondents to consider their WTP to achieve reductions in the risks of those outcomes (Loomes, 2004). This raises challenging problems for stated-preference work since it is well known that many respondents are insufficiently sensitive to information about small changes in small risks, and it may well prove impossible to find any satisfactory way of communicating the risk information.

As an alternative, 'certainty' scenarios might be used and valued using willingness to accept (WTA) rather than the more traditionally used WTP. The principle underlying WTA is that if an individual contemplates some adverse event, the loss of welfare could be offset by the welfare generated by some increase in wealth. Clearly, this does not necessarily apply to more severe levels of harm, such as death, where no amount of money may adequately compensate for the loss (and where respondents may be offended that such a comparison is sought at all). However, for many crime outcomes, it may be possible to argue that there are finite sums that would offset the experience (or at least, to explore how far that may be the case).

Rather than elicit valuations directly, a contingent ranking exercise offers an indirect way of eliciting monetary values. The contingent ranking approach asks respondents to compare alternatives, each involving various differences along the kind of dimensions outlined in the appendix. The general idea is that the relative weights assigned to different levels along the different dimensions can be inferred from the sets of rankings. If various sums of money can also be included, it should in principle be possible to infer the rate of trade-off between money and any level along any dimension. This class of choice-based techniques is believed to mimic the kinds of choices people might be expected to make in real life.

In the event that we are not confident that respondents are sufficiently sensitive to risk, the relativities obtained from contingent rankings may allow us to 'chain' the values for more serious outcomes (which we cannot plausibly obtain from WTP questions about preventing the *certainty* of those outcomes) to values for less serious outcomes that may be amenable to WTP (and WTA) questions using certainties rather than risks. However, the statistical procedures for inferring the various trade-offs often make somewhat restrictive assumptions about the underlying structure of people's preferences, and a large number of choices might be required to obtain the minimum amount of information to enable the estimation procedure to be implemented.

In a recent WTP study in crime, Cohen *et al.* (2004) found an implied WTP per avoided crime well in excess of previous estimates based on victim costs, and suggest that the difference may be in part due to their study incorporating costs that have been overlooked in previous studies, including the anxieties people have about anticipated crime. The study finds an implied WTP for avoiding one burglary of \$25 000, avoiding one rape or sexual assault of \$237 000 and avoiding one murder of \$9 700 000. However, these differences may well be driven to a significant extent by the different frequencies of these crimes, since the mean willingness to pay for a 10% reduction in each of these crimes was very similar; \$104, \$127, and \$146, respectively. The results do give weight to the notion that the fear of crime substantially reduces well-being, but the dominance of probabilities on the final WTP figures may be thought to raise serious doubts about the reliability of the results.

More generally, there has been much discussion in the literature about potential sources of bias in WTP/WTA studies and we will not rehearse them in any detail here (see Carson *et al.*, 2001). Some of the more pervasive problems, and ones that will be relevant to the context of crime, are: *warm-glow effects*, which occur when the respondent feels some moral obligation towards the scenario being valued (Diamond and Hausman, 1993); *embedding effects*, which occur when the respondent reacts to a good's general symbolic meaning instead of to the specific levels of provision described (Mitchell and Carson, 1989); and *scope effects*, which occur when responses are insensitive to the quantity of the good being valued. Some of these biases have been reduced by improved research design (Arrow *et al.*, 1993) but scope effects, for example, have proved to be particularly pervasive. Moreover, even if studies could perfectly replicate a market, there are questions about the degree to which the market itself is free of the some of these biases.

Non-monetary valuations

The aim here is to elicit the values of the outcome descriptions relative to one another. A subsequent task is then to 'peg' these to some monetary value(s). The valuations are relative to two anchor points. In the health-state valuation literature, death and full health are typically used as the anchor points, and given the value of zero and one, respectively. The upper anchor in the context of crime valuation should be the combination of no problems across all dimensions, with no mention of crime. However, it is not clear whether the lower anchor should be death caused by crime, or death with no cause specified. The latter will match better with the upper anchor, but if death by crime is perceived as worse than death by, say illness, or by accident, then this should be taken into account.

Direct valuations for crime outcomes could be elicited using the standard gamble (SG) method or the time trade-off (TTO) method (Dolan, 2000). The basic SG asks the respondent to choose between the certainty of an intermediate health state and an alternative treatment with two probabilistic outcomes, one of which is better than the certain outcome and one of which is worse. The probabilities are changed until the respondent is indifferent between the two scenarios. The basic TTO asks the respondent to choose between two alternatives, one is to live for a defined period of time in poor health and then die, and the second is to live for a shorter period of time in full health and then die. The length of time in full health is changed until the respondent is indifferent between the two scenarios.

There are then ways to express the duration of a given outcome. One alternative is to make the duration of the outcome the same as that of the entire scenario, e.g. 'you will experience outcome *i* for *t* years, and then die'. Since many crime outcomes will last for much shorter durations than the life expectancy of a typical respondent, this may be difficult for respondents to take at face value and engage in. Therefore, the second alternative is to make the duration of the outcome shorter than the overall duration of the scenario, e.g. 'you will experience outcome *i* for *t* years (or *m* months), and then survive to your naturally expected age of death in full health'.

However, there are two issues associated with this. Firstly, suppose the duration of the outcome is set very short relative to the time horizon, such as when an outcome will last for one month during the next 10 years. If a respondent to a TTO question is willing to trade off more than one month at the end of the 10 years, then (in the absence of discounting) the outcome in question will have a negative value, implying that it is worse than being dead. Likewise, if a respondent to a SG question is willing to take more than a 0.008 risk of death, then the outcome will also be valued as if it were worse than being dead. Secondly, the valuations will not be anchored at 0 for dead, and there needs to be an additional exercise to provide this link.

A further issue arises when respondents are faced with outcomes that involve relatively mild losses, which they acknowledge are worse than full health but for which they are also unwilling to trade off any survival or take any risk of death. One way to address this issue is to value these mild states using a more severe outcome that is preferred to death as the bottom anchor in the TTO and SG elicitations (rather than using death, as in the basic formats described above). If this intermediate outcome is then valued against full health and death, the results of this elicitation can be used to 'chain' the results obtained for all the other outcomes to the standard 0 to 1 (death to full health) scale. This chaining method results in values for mild outcomes that are less than the value for full health. The problem with chaining is that it may introduce an additional source of noise and error. An alternative, which is to set an intermediate additional anchor (rather than replacing the bottom anchor), may be preferable in the case of crime, but again will need to be investigated in terms of whether it means the same to all respondents.

It is possible to elicit non-monetary valuations indirectly by asking respondents to rank a number of different outcomes (McCabe *et al.*, 2006), or by asking them to make a series of choices between different pairs of outcomes, as in discrete choice experiments. The data from the ranking or discrete choice exercise are then analysed in ways that allow cardinal values at the group level to be generated from ordinal data at the individual level. Where the descriptive system does not include money, the results can be anchored to full health and being dead by including dead as one of the states in the discrete choice or ranking exercise. Where the system does include the monetary dimension, the results could be reported in terms of monetary value per one-level change in each dimension.

DISCUSSION

In order to determine how best to allocate resources that seek to reduce the impact of crime on society, we need to describe the important consequences of crime and the fear of crime in ways that facilitate the practical collection of epidemiological data and the elicitation of robust valuation data. As well as the description and valuation issues identified in this paper, there are a number of other methodological and practical challenges we face in trying to develop a measure of public safety. The effects of crime and the fear associated with it can be felt not only by individual victims, but also by their families, friends and colleagues. There may well be similar externalities associated with ill-health, but they would seem to be more pronounced in the context of crime, particularly in relation to murder and sexual assaults. This suggests that samples need to be drawn from a wide range of sources and not just from victims of crime.

The effects can also be experienced many times, as in the case of repeat victimisation (or just by vividly recalling the episode as some PTSD sufferers do). On the basis of existing evidence, it is difficult to predict the direction for multiple victimisations. Additional injuries might have an increasing marginal effect, but the UK criminal compensation tariff seems to take the opposite view, where the most severe injury is taken as a reference point and additional injuries are included at reduced rates. Therefore, we need to elicit valuations from those with repeated (real or perceived) exposure to crime.

There is also the need to consider the effect that the criminal justice system may have on how people react to criminal victimisation. There are parallels here with health, where the process of health care may affect people's response to treatment, but the effects would again seem to be more pronounced in the context of crime, where the sentence given to the perpetrator of the crime can have an important effect on how well the victim deals with the crime. This is recognised by the increasing interest in 'restorative justice', which brings victims and offenders together in order to allow victims greater voice in the criminal justice system.

Once robust measures of the individual losses in well-being from crime and the fear of crime have been developed, there will be the need to determine the social value of these losses. There are again strong parallels to health here, where the development and use of QALYs has led to questions about whether it is appropriate for policy purposes to assume that 'a QALY is a QALY is a QALY', irrespective of the characteristics of its recipient. While this represents the default position adopted by the National Institute for Health and Clinical Excellence (NICE) in its evaluation of healthcare technologies, there is ongoing empirical research into its validity. Developing an equity-weighted measure of public safety will be particularly important given the very unequal distribution of the effects of crime across society. While most of us can expect to get ill and need health care at some point in our lives, crime is heavily concentrated in certain geographical areas, and within those areas on certain households and individuals (Pease, 2001).

But the primary need is to develop a robust measure of public safety. In short, what is required is an 'EQ-5D for crime'. We have recently co-ordinated an ESRC-funded seminar series on 'Crime, insecurity and well-being: an economic approach', which has many parallels to the EuroQol group in that it has brought together academics from a range of disciplines, and policy makers, to consider how best to describe and value the losses in well-being from crime in order to inform public sector resource-allocation decisions. Alan attended some of the earlier seminars and we believe he would be pleased to hear that we are planning to take the empirical research forward through grant proposals.

ACKNOWLEDGEMENTS

We would like to acknowledge Alan Williams for inspiring our (academic) interest in crime in the first place. Many of the ideas in the paper are the result of working with Graham Loomes and Tessa Peasgood on two Home Office reports on the intangible costs of crime and the fear of crime. We have also been influenced by discussions as part of an ESRC seminar series on crime, insecurity and well-being, where the input of Simon Moore and Joanna Shapland has been particularly helpful. The usual disclaimers apply.

REFERENCES

Adler M (2004) Fear assessment: cost–benefit analysis and the pricing of fear and anxiety. *Chicago-Kent Law Review* **79**: 977–1053.

Arrow K, Solow R, Portney PR *et al.* (1993) Report of the NOAA Panel on Contingent Valuation. *Federal Register* **58**: 4601–14.

Atkinson G, Dubourg R and Mourato S (2004) Market-based approaches to valuing non-market economic impacts. Paper presented at First ESRC Seminar on Crime, insecurity, and well-being: an economic approach. Sheffield: Centre for Well-being in Public Policy, University of Sheffield.

Bannister J and Fyfe H (2001) Introduction: fear and the city, *Urban Studies* **38**: 807–13.

Carson RT, Flores N and Meade NF (2001) Contingent valuation: controversies and evidence. *Environmental and Resource Economics* **19**: 173–210.

Clark AE and Oswald AJ (2002) A simple statistical method for measuring how life events affect happiness. *International Journal of Epidemiology* **31**: 1139–44.

Cohen MA, Rust RT, Steen S and Tidd ST (2004) Willingness-to-pay for crime control programs. *Criminology* **42**: 89–109.

Denkers A and Winkel F (1997) Crime victims' well being and fear in a prospective and longitudinal study. *International Review of Victimology* **5**: 141–62.

Diamond PA and Hausman J (1993) On contingent valuation measurement of nonuse values. In: Hausman J (ed.) *Contingent Valuation: a critical assessment*. Amsterdam: North Holland, pp. 3–38.

Ditton J, Bannister J, Gilchrist E and Farrall S (1999) Afraid or angry? Recalibrating the 'fear' of crime. *International Review of Victimology* **6**: 83–99.

Dolan P (2000) The measurement of health-related quality of life for use in resource allocation decisions. In: Culyer AJ and Newhouse J (eds) *Health Care, Handbook of Health Economics*, Amsterdam: Elsevier, pp. 1723–60.

Dolan P, Loomes G, Peasgood T and Tsuchiya A (2005) Estimating the intangible victim costs of crime. *British Journal of Criminology* **45**: 958–76.

Dolan P, Netten A, Shapland J and Tsuchiya A (2007) Towards a preference-based measure of the impact on well-being of crime and the fear of crime. *International Review of Victimology* (in press).

Dolan P and Peasgood T (2006) Estimating the economic and social costs of the fear of crime. *British Journal of Criminology* **47**: 121– 32.

Dubourg R, Hamed J and Thorns J (2005) *The Economic and Social Costs of Crime against Individuals and Households 2003–4*. Home Office Online Report, 30/05. Available at: www.homeoffice.gov.uk/rds/pdfs05/rdsolr3005.pdf

Farrall S and Gadd D (2004) *Evaluating Crime Fears: a research note on a pilot study to improve the measurement of the 'fear of crime' as a performance indicator*. Unpublished paper, Department of Criminology, Keele University.

Hale C (1995) Fear of crime: a review of the literature. *International Review of Victimology* **4**: 79–150.

HM Treasury (2003) *The Green Book: appraisal and evaluation in central government.* London: The Stationery Office. Available at: http://greenbook.treasury.gov.uk/

Loomes G (2004) *Valuing Reductions in the Risk of Being a Victim of Crime: the 'willingness to pay' approach to valuing the 'intangible costs' of crime.* Paper presented at the First ESRC Seminar on Crime, Insecurity, and Well-being: an economic approach. Centre for Well-being in Public Policy, University of Sheffield, January 2004.

Lynch AK and Rasmussen DW (2001) Measuring the impact of crime on house prices. *Applied Economics* **33**: 1981–9.

McCabe C, Brazier J, Gilks P *et al.* (2006) Estimating population cardinal health state valuation models from individual ordinal (rank) health state preference data. *Journal of Health Economics* **25**: 418–31.

Mitchell RC and Carson RT (1989) *Using Surveys to Value Public Goods: the contingent valuation method.* Washington DC: Resources for the Future (Johns Hopkins University Press).

Pease K (2001) Distributive justice and crime, *European Journal on Criminal Policy and Research* **9**: 413–25.

Semmens N (2004) *The Intangible Costs of Crime: why the fear of crime causes us a problem?* Paper presented at the Second ESRC Seminar on Crime, Insecurity, and Well-being: an economic approach. Centre for Well-being in Public Policy, University of Sheffield, January 2004.

Shapland J and Hall M (2004) *What do we Know about the Effects of Crime on Victims?* Paper presented at the Second ESRC Seminar on Crime, Insecurity, and Well-being: an economic approach. Centre for Well-being in Public Policy, University of Sheffield, January 2004.

Shapland J, Willmore J and Duff P (1985) *Victims in the Criminal Justice System.* Aldershot: Gower.

Williams A (2005) Discovering the QALY, or how Rachel Rosser changed my life. In: Oliver A (ed.) *Personal Histories in Health Research.* London: The Nuffield Trust, pp. 191–206.

Winkel F (1998) Fear of crime and criminal victimization: testing a theory of psychological incapacitation of the 'stressor' based on downward comparison processes. *British Journal of Criminology* **38**: 473–84.

Winkielman P, Schwarz N and Belli RF (1998) The role of ease of retrieval and attribution in memory judgments: judging your memory as worse despite recalling more events. *Psychological Science* **9**: 124–6.

APPENDIX: EXAMPLE CRIME STATE CLASSIFICATION SYSTEM

We will describe some states that you may find yourself in because of crime. When we say 'because of crime', this can be caused by being a victim of a criminal offence, or by witnessing a criminal act first hand, or by simply hearing about a crime on television. Also, the crime can be violent and cause injuries, or non-violent and only involve loss in property. Such experiences will affect people in different ways. Here we are just describing the effects of the experience.

The first is *physical health problems*
A No physical health problems
B Mild problems with physical health (e.g. difficulty running fast; limited hearing)
C Moderate problems with physical health (e.g. use a stick to walk around; moderate intermittent pain)
D Extreme problems with physical health (e.g. use a wheelchair; severe pain)

The second one is *mental health problems*
A No mental health problems
B Mild problems with mental health (e.g. feel somewhat anxious; mild depression)
C Moderate problems with mental health (e.g. occasional anxiousness; persistent mild irritability)
D Extreme problems with mental health (e.g. severe depression; hallucination)

The third is *constraints on behaviour*
A No constraints on behaviour (e.g. I can do what I want and go where I want)
B Mild constraints on behaviour (e.g. there are some constraints on what I do and there are a few places I cannot go)
C Moderate problems with control (e.g. there are many things I cannot do and a number of places I cannot go)
D Extreme problems with control (e.g. I can do hardly anything I would like to and there are very few places I can go)

The fourth is *how you relate to others*
A No relational problems
B Mild relational problems (e.g. feel that other people will let me down)
C Moderate relational problems (e.g. mistrust of strangers; unease when out and about in the community)
D Extreme relational problems (e.g. mistrust of intimate family members; feel completely alone all the time)

The fifth is *how vulnerable you feel*
A No vulnerability problems
B Mild vulnerability because of crime (e.g. sometimes just worry about getting things wrong)
C Moderate vulnerability problems because of crime (e.g. occasionally worry that everything could be lost)
D Extreme vulnerability problems because of crime (e.g. feel strongly that something is bound to go seriously wrong and nothing can be done about it)

CHAPTER 13

Discussion of Paul Dolan and Aki Tsuchiya's paper: 'The measurement and valuation of public safety'

. . . Martin Buxton

As the authors suggest, this paper would almost certainly have pleased Alan Williams in the way it takes the concept of the QALY and begins to explore how it, or something like it, might be applied to an area of public spending other than health care. Alan's early involvement with the Treasury meant that he was well aware of the need to consider value for money in all aspects of the public sector. However, I suggest, that he, like me, would have wanted to contextualise this work as part of a wider, more ambitious agenda that could lead to a methodology for comparing cost-effectiveness across a variety of areas of public sector spending.

As it stands, the preliminary descriptive system proposed by Dolan and Tsuchiya (and set out in the Appendix to their paper) for what Alan Williams called their SALY (safety-adjusted life year) bears a strong family resemblance to the EQ-5D health-related quality of life descriptive system.* It sets out to provide a classification system that 'allows the different attributes of well-being that are affected by crime to be combined into overall "crime states"'. In this paper setting out early ideas, many of the details of the valuation process are still unclear. They do however propose a familiar process for the valuation of states relative both to each other and to the anchor points of, at the top end, no problems related to any of the dimensions characterising the effects of crime and, at the other end, death. They suggest that this may have to be 'a natural death', to allow for the likely possibility that death as a result of crime is perceived as worse than death by illness or accident.

The precise relationship of this new measure to the EQ-5D (or other existing QALY measures used in health) is unclear. Indeed it is not explicit

* For a description of the EQ-5D system, and its development, see for example Williams (1997).

whether the authors assume that it should have a precise relationship to a QALY. There appears to be a considerable degree of 'content' overlap between this and the EQ-5D, but without a clear indication, for example, of which dimensions of the EQ-5D will be covered by the first proposed dimension of 'physical health' in this new instrument, or how the 'mental health problems' dimension relates to the EQ-5D dimension of 'anxiety/ depression'. It is curious, but probably relatively unimportant, that Dolan and Tsuchiya suggest four levels for each of the dimensions, when the EQ-5D instrument currently uses three and the EuroQol group is busy attempting to remodel the instrument with five levels (Kind and Macran, 2002). More fundamentally, it is unclear to me whether the four dimensions of 'mental health problems', 'constraints on behaviour', 'relationship to others' and 'feelings of vulnerability' are conceptually sufficiently separable to make a subsequent valuation process meaningful. Other readers would no doubt identify additional concerns of detail.

However, this is essentially an 'ideas' paper, in which much of the detail is not yet finalised, and my main focus therefore is not on the detail but on the bigger, and ultimately more important, picture. Of course, I can see a real value for the Home Office in what the authors propose: it would provide a useful measure of effectiveness against which to compare different policies to reduce the extent, or effect, of crime. But in the bigger schema, how would a cost per QALY from a health-sector investment be compared with a cost per SALY from a Home Office investment? Would not Alan, who was rarely daunted by the magnitude of a task he saw as important, have wanted this instrument alongside his much loved QALY to be capable of addressing this comparison?

Essentially the EQ-5D provides a means to record and value the adjustment to length of life due to *health-related* quality of life. It has long been criticised by some economists because it may not adequately represent individual preferences for health outcomes (for example, Mehrez and Gafni (1999)) and by others in that it does not directly address all the factors, such as information, that would appear in an individual's utility function (for example Protiere *et al.*, 2004). Rather it provides a partial measure focusing on the impact of changes in *health outcomes*. The focus on *health* outcomes is most often justified in terms of its use in helping to estimate the effectiveness of *health* interventions funded predominantly from *health service* budgets.

Dolan and Tsuchiya now offer us the potential for a new quality adjustment reflecting security or the non-pecuniary effects of crime. Rather than a SALY – a security-adjusted life year – it is perhaps more useful to think of it as a *crime-related* QALY. Again the argument for this focus is that for the Home Office this measure potentially offers a method to show how interventions within its control can change quality of life. Essentially it provides another sectoral and partial QALY.

It does not involve a great flight of imagination to see the possibilities for other partial or sectoral QALY measures. It is easy to imagine an *environment-related* QALY or an *education/opportunities-related* QALY, which might provide broadly equivalent measures for other areas of public spending. But before we get to that point – indeed arguably before Dolan and Tsuchiya go further with crime-related SALY – we need to consider how these various QALYs should relate to each other.

One possible model is to actively encourage the development of a series of non-overlapping sectoral descriptors of the way in which, and extent to which, quality of life is diminished by sectoral factors – health, crime, environment, education and opportunities, etc. Each would need to be scaled (directly or indirectly) in a similar way. Tentatively, I would suggest that might be from the absence of any diminution of quality of life with respect to that 'sector' (value 1) to 'natural death' (value 0). If they are to be used together it would be desirable that the scales did not overlap, and so the SALY here would not include any descriptors or dimensions of health that appeared in, or were already covered by, the health-related QALY. (In principle it would be possible to allow for some common dimensions, if described identically.) An additional partial QALY could be developed for any set of 'sectoral factors' not hitherto covered, so clearly an initial task might be to consider what the full range of sectoral QALYs might look like.

This development also opens up the opportunity to consider what characteristics of the process, by which services are delivered, contribute to individual and collective well-being, and to include these in a component of the super-QALY. For example reduced waiting times for appointments with the health system (even if they have no impact on outcomes) values, like faster police response times, appear to have a real value to the public (Cave *et al.*, 1993).

Together they would enable us to describe, measure and value what I would call a '*super-QALY*'* – a super-QALY being equivalent to a year of life undiminished by limitations in any major aspect of life (or at least on any contributing QALY instrument). A super-QALY would thus have to combine adjustments for limitations on any scale, so that there would need to be a cross-sectoral relative valuation exercise to establish how values for one factor compare to another. In principle, a cross-sectoral exercise could seek to set values for each of all the combined states that the system describes.

Of course in practice, the partial QALYs which contribute to the super-QALY are not exclusively produced by or attributable to any one sector of the economy or public sector spending. It would in principle be possible to generate any type of QALY in any context. Thus for example, crime reduction might well generate improvements that would be measured on the health-related, as well as the crime-related, QALY scales. Similarly health

* I am aware that others have used the term super-QALY in different ways, particularly to describe an equity-weighted QALY, as for example by Anand (1999). I would contest that my use of the term is more appropriate and consistent with both the correct and common usage of the adjective, but I confess bias in this respect.

interventions for children might well generate health-related and education/ opportunities-related QALYs. Full-blown evaluations of an intervention could consider all dimensions; more limited evaluations could focus on the most important and relevant sectoral scale.

Obviously such a broader vision needs to be thoroughly debated. There would clearly be those advocates of cost–benefit analysis, who would argue that it is all unnecessary and that it just emphasises the need to use monetary valuations of changes, without complex, intermediate multidimensional scaling. There would be others who might argue that we should proceed on a piecemeal basis sector by sector, as implicitly accepted in this paper, because that way useful progress can be made more quickly and the pursuit of the 'holy grail' will only stand in the way of more modest but valuable progress. There will be those existing users of health-related QALYs who will appreciate that such an approach has important implications for our existing measures, and may resist rethinking aspects of them. For example, the concept of a natural death, introduced in the Dolan and Tsuchiya paper, brings into question what has been implicitly assumed, for example in the EQ-5D valuation exercises, but potentially offers a system that can much more readily reflect what many would believe, that valuable quality of life can be gained by allowing death to take place in a more natural way or in a more natural environment – the belated recognition of which would receive a cheer from the hospice and homecare movements.

This brief discussion is not the place to attempt to anticipate that vigorous debate, but the Dolan and Tsuchiya paper provides an excellent incentive, and an urgent reason, to begin such a debate. I would not be so bold as to claim I know what position Alan Williams would have taken, but I'm confident he would have enjoyed, encouraged and taken an active part in that debate, and he would not have been daunted by the magnitude of the potential research agenda it might create.

REFERENCES

Anand P (1999) QALYS and the integration of claims in health-care rationing, *Health Care Analysis* 7: 239–53.

Cave M, Burningham D, Buxton M *et al.* (1993) *The Valuation of Changes in Quality in the Public Services.* Report prepared for HM Treasury by Brunel University. London: HMSO.

Kind P and Macran S (2002) *Levelling the Playing Field: increasing the number of response categories in EQ-5D.* Proceedings of the 19th Plenary Meeting of the EuroQol Group, University of York, September 2002. http://gs1.q4matics.com/euroqol_zoek_test/DocumentBekijken.rbm?DocID=110117&KlantID=125 (accessed 9 March 2007).

Mehrez A and Gafni A (1989) Quality adjusted life years (QALYs), utility theory and healthy years equivalent. *Medical Decision Making* **9**: 142–9.

Protiere C, Donaldson C, Luchini S *et al.* (2004) The impact of information on non-health attributes on willingness to pay for multiple health care programmes, *Social Science and Medicine* **58**: 1257–69.

Williams A (1997) The measurement and valuation of health: a chronicle. In: Culyer AJ and Maynard AK (eds). *Being Reasonable about the Economics of Health.* Cheltenham: Edward Elgar Publishing Limited, pp. 136–75.

Index